healthy choices, healthy children

A GUIDE TO RAISING FIT, HAPPY KIDS

Lori S. Brizee, MS, RD, CSP

with Sue Schumann Warner

PARACLETE PRESS
BREWSTER, MASSACHUSETTS

Healthy Choices, Healthy Children: A Guide to Raising Fit, Happy Kids
Copyright © 2011 by Lori S. Brizee and Sue Schumann Warner
ISBN 978-1-55725-924-0

My Plate graphic as it appears on page 18 used by permission of the USDA Center for Nutrition Policy and Promotion (CNPP).

Library of Congress Cataloging-in-Publication Data

Brizee, Lori S.

  Healthy choices, healthy children : a guide to raising fit, happy kids / Lori S. Brizee, Sue Schumann Warner.

      p. cm.

  Summary: "This easy-to-use guide provides essential tools for raising well-nourished, active children who will make lifelong healthy choices. Engaging, practical, and filled with quick tips, this is a must read for the busy parent trying to navigate the challenging world of kids and food. An ideal book for parents, schools, churches, and community groups. Recipes are included"—Provided by publisher.

  ISBN 978-1-55725-924-0 (pbk.)

  1. Children—Nutrition. 2. Physical fitness for children. 3. Children—Health and hygiene. I. Schumann Warner, Sue. II. Title.

  RJ206.B756 2011

  618.92—dc23   2011022630

10 9 8 7 6 5 4 3 2 1

Published by Paraclete Press
Brewster, Massachusetts
www.paracletepress.com
Printed in the United States of America

I dedicate this book to my husband, Bob, and my kids, Suzanne and Michael, who have given me inspiration throughout my life and career and have encouraged me in every step of writing this book.

—Lori S. Brizee

Contents

Part Four Putting It into Practice

Appendices

Introduction

AS A NUTRITIONIST FOR NEARLY THIRTY YEARS, primarily in pediatrics, I've seen firsthand the growing need for families to take a more active role in teaching their children about healthy living and healthy eating. And as a community we must support families and caregivers by providing them with up-to-date information and realistic suggestions that are easily incorporated into their busy and complicated lives. *Healthy Choices, Healthy Children* is my attempt to create such a resource. This book can help us reverse the rising tide of obesity and raise children who are physically fit, healthy, and well nourished.

Of course, we and our children are far more than just physical beings. In order for any of us to truly be "successful" as human beings, we need to develop in mind, body, and spirit. If we focus on just one area for our child, we will stifle the opportunity for growth in others. An extremely intelligent child may excel beyond his age level in every subject and read at a college level by age twelve. But if he is eating poorly, getting no physical activity, and has not developed social skills, he will have a very difficult life in spite of his great talents. Or we may have a child who is an amazing athlete—definitely on the road to a soccer scholarship for college. If this child does not work hard in school, develop good communication skills, and learn compassion for others, she will have a less than joyful life.

There are many references in the Bible and other sacred writings to raising our children—we are told over and over to teach them and to be examples for them. Our children and grandchildren are a blessing to us—we want to love them unconditionally. We want to encourage their strengths and help build their self-esteem and character.

Every child has strengths and weaknesses—physically, mentally, and spiritually. Some are visible and some are not. Children with visible differences—birth defects that affect their appearance, accidents that result in disfigurement, as well as obesity—are stigmatized. Children face discrimination and prejudice every day when they "look different." Research suggests that parents may also treat these children differently than they do their more "normal-appearing" children. Parents who have children with any characteristic that society views as outside of normal and healthy have a hard road.

As a community of caring people, we need to teach our kids to treat each other as children of God. As adults, we need to evaluate our prejudices and figure out where they come from. I firmly believe that we need to ask ourselves, every day, how we can truly love our neighbors— that includes our families, our friends (and our children's friends), our business associates, our acquaintances, the people in the next town ... you get the picture.

I see the misery that many kids deal with because of their weight. My heart breaks as I hear stories of teasing, discrimination, and overall poor treatment because of a child's obesity—especially when it comes from adults, whom we would expect to be more understanding. Our kids live in a stressful world—and they handle stress in a variety of different ways. Some of them overeat, others don't eat well at all, some take up other self-destructive behaviors—drugs, alcohol, and on and on. Our job is to affirm our kids, to let them know they are loved, and to guide them in healthy lifestyle habits.

My hope is that this book will help parents, grandparents, teachers, and other adults better understand how we can change our environment, our ways of eating, and our activity to decrease the epidemic of obesity in children. There is much to be done to reverse this trend. It has to start with individuals and families who care and expand to the people making decisions about our food supply and community environment.

So, how can we help our children who have weight issues? By truly caring for our children and teaching them that they are loved by God—and by us—we can help them to love themselves and be the people they were meant to be. Their worth has nothing to do with their weight.

However, we want our kids to be healthy, so we definitely want them to be at a healthy weight. We need to focus on choosing healthy foods, limiting less healthy ones, getting physical activity, and cutting back on those sit-down activities—TV, videos, computer games. We want to do this simply because it is the right thing to do for all our kids, not just our overweight children. We want to do this because we love our children and know that it is best to work on being physically healthy.

How do we bring in the mental and spiritual aspects of being healthy? We want to stimulate our children's minds—talk with them, spend time with them, read with them, talk about current events, take them to cultural events—and set limits, such as doing homework and reading before kicking back to watch TV or play a video game. We want to be involved in their schools as much as is possible and appropriate, getting to know their teachers. By helping our kids advance their mental skills, we are helping them get ready to be functional adults.

The spiritual is where many of us fall short. We may not be involved in an organized church or faith practice. That does not mean that we do not have a spiritual component to our lives—that part of us that resonates deep inside when we see a beautiful sunset, admire the intricacies of a small wildflower, or hear beautiful music. That part of us that wells up with joy when our child gives us an unsolicited hug, draws us a picture, or brings us a gift. That part of us that cries inside when our child is hurting or is left out.

Our spirit is the part of us that enables us to feel both joy and sadness. We want to build our own spiritual strength—maybe we read the Bible and pray, learn to meditate, or practice yoga. Maybe we reflect on creation and nature while we take a walk. Maybe we go to a museum to see great art, or listen to our favorite music. We need to do things for ourselves that are "good for the soul," that rejuvenate our hectic lives. We have to allow ourselves the time to just "be"—by allowing our spirit to come to the surface, we are role models for our children.

If you are not already doing so, begin giving thanks before your meals; we are all grateful that we have food to eat. We are teaching our children a wonderful spiritual practice when we take time to express our thankfulness for what we have. Another thing we can do is spend some time with our children at bedtime either praying or just reviewing the day—talk about the wind in the trees, the kid who got hurt at recess, the way we felt when certain things happened. This is a great way to get a read on how your child's spirit is doing—is she sad, joyful, frustrated? It is also a way to say that you love her, and she is important and worthy.

We cannot spend all our time on just one aspect of our lives—if we do, we will be terribly unbalanced and incomplete. The parent who feels his child is a failure if he does not go to college is similar to the parent who feels his child is a failure because he is morbidly obese—neither child is a "failure." We may encourage our child to go to college and encourage our child to be healthy, but our love is not complete if it is conditional.

Why are our children becoming obese in epidemic proportions? Today, one in three children and adolescents is overweight and one in six is obese—an increase of almost 340 percent since the 1960s. This statistic is alarming, as eight out of ten obese teens become obese adults. The health implications are staggering: increased type 2 diabetes, hypertension, high cholesterol, cardiovascular disease, breast and prostate cancers, gall bladder disease, arthritis, depression . . . the list goes on and on. If we think we have a healthcare crisis now, just wait a few years!

This is not only a problem in the United States—children in the United Kingdom are becoming obese almost twice as fast as those in the United States. Everywhere that food is abundant, obesity is on the rise. This is a global public health crisis.

Obesity-related health problems such as diabetes, hypertension, and heart disease may not develop during childhood, but they surely will during adulthood, and at much earlier ages than in years past, when obesity in children and young adults was far less prevalent.

Why are so many children overweight or obese? Increased screen time (TV, computer games, videos), high-calorie fast food and convenience food, sugared drinks, less outdoor "play" time, and eating on the run are just a few of the culprits. Add in high food costs for healthy foods compared to the low costs for processed foods containing high levels of sugar, salt, and fat, super-sized portions at restaurants and in packaged foods, and the demise of the family meal, and you've got a recipe for disaster.

Yet I've seen the amazing transformations that occur when kids—and their families—adopt simple, healthy eating habits.

There is hope.

Consider Bill, one of my young adult weight management clients. As a child, he was one of those "big and tall" kids; in middle school, he gained weight rapidly. When he entered college, he weighed around 300 pounds, and he ballooned to more than 400 pounds after graduating.

Bill was motivated to decrease his weight—he knew it was making it hard for him to become employed. He realized that a combination of emotional eating around the time of his parents' divorce, when he was ten years old, and then poor eating habits in his teen years were among many factors in his weight gain. He is now making great strides in managing his weight and improving his health through sound nutrition and physical activity.

Parents want their kids to be as healthy as possible. Many of us grew up eating a lot of "junk foods" ourselves and never learned how to eat a truly healthy diet. Many say that we don't like fruits and vegetables and just figure that our kids won't either. Many of us are too tired at the end of the day—understandably so—to prepare a "sit down" meal.

Healthy Choices, Healthy Children addresses these concerns and others and provides the simple, easy-to-use tools you need to raise fit, well-nourished kids.

Healthy kids start with healthy parents. If you are a parent, don't be surprised if you choose to make changes in your own lifestyle and health, so that you can help your kids develop lifelong healthy habits.

And remember—by picking up this book, reading the chapters, and putting the principles into practice, you're off to a good start!

Part One

Back to Basics

The "Hows" of Eating

KIDS CAN BE A PAIN AT THE DINNER TABLE! They say "yuck" to the wonderful food you've prepared. They poke each other, spill their milk, whine, and complain . . . until you say, "See why I feed them by themselves!" When my kids were young, we started a "three strikes and you're out" rule. The kids got a strike for saying "yuck," whining or complaining, feeding the dog from the table, fighting or arguing with each other, or any other dinner table misdemeanor.

If they got three strikes, they had to leave the room—meal over! Neither of them ever got three strikes more than once or twice (they both got to strike two lots of times). It became a game—sometimes if they did something especially aggravating (like punching each other or spitting something out) we'd say, "That's strikes one and two!" They didn't really want to leave the table, so they'd shape up.

Sometimes, after an especially stressful day, I'd say, "I want three strikes, so I can just go to my room!" That always got some laughs.

● ● ● ● ● ● ● ● ● ● ● ● ●

Life is busy!

Kids' schedules . . . parents' schedules . . . single parenting . . . blended families . . . jobs . . . sports . . . When is there time to think about how—when and where—our children are eating? It's tough enough just to get them fed!

If you've picked up this book, you want to make changes—provide a healthy foundation for your children's health now and in the future—and in reading it, you've *already* started.

Keep on reading, to see how a few simple changes in how our families eat can make a huge difference.

When to eat

Give kids three meals and two to three snacks a day, with at least two and no more than four hours between each eating time. (This is a good guide for all of us, from toddlers to adults!)

How our kids eat is just as important as *what* they eat.

Children who are overweight or underweight are frequently grazers—like the petite child with a "fragile appetite" who sips on juice or milk and snacks on little bits of food throughout the day, taking the edge off her appetite. She never eats enough to meet her needs and as a result is underweight.

Another child with a "hearty appetite" will graze throughout the day, taking in more than he needs, ending up overweight.

We can help our kids learn their "hunger and fullness cues" by offering them food five to six times per day—three meals and two to three snacks. Kids can't meet all their nutritional needs in three meals per day, so snacks are important. If a child has a minimum of two hours to a maximum of four hours between eating times, she has time to develop an appetite without becoming overly hungry, and she will be more apt to eat the foods offered to her at meals until she feels comfortably full.

If she is nibbling on crackers or sipping juice throughout the day, she will be far more likely to turn up her nose at a meal you've prepared, and far less likely to eat the foods that truly nourish her.

Where to eat

Children (and adults) should eat at a table—without the TV on.

I recently spoke at a parents' group and discussed the importance of having "eating places," such as the kitchen table. One mom said she often eats over the kitchen sink. The day before, she gave her two-and-a-half-year-old a sandwich at the table, but he said he wanted to eat like Mommy does . . . so he brought a chair over to the sink and ate his sandwich there. His observation was a revelation to her—and to the rest of us. Children do as we *do* and not as we *say*.

What we eat is important, but *how* we eat is equally important. If we eat while we are doing something else, we'll often keep eating until the food is gone; if we *just* eat, however—and don't combine it with other activities—we usually eat what we are truly hungry for.

Take a minute and think about your (and your family's) eating habits and see if there are times when you eat mindlessly—in front of the TV, while driving in the car, reading, doing homework. Ask yourself how you can increase "mindful" eating and decrease the "mindless" munching.

Try starting a household "rule" (for kids *and* parents) that all eating and drinking is done at the table without the TV on. This doesn't restrict what or how much you and your kids eat but definitely helps to prevent "mindless" eating. (As a side benefit, it keeps your house cleaner!) After just a week, you'll notice a big difference in your eating habits.

Go a step further and make eating times truly special. If you are eating take-out food, put it on plates. Maybe even put flowers on the table or light a candle. Sit down together and enjoy your food. Wait until everyone is seated to start eating. Mealtime is a great time to practice giving thanks—for the food you will be eating and for those who grew and prepared it. One simple prayer is: "For health and strength and daily food, we give thanks." Another is: "Lord, make us truly grateful for the blessings of this day." (You do not have to be religious to acknowledge that having food to eat several times each day is a privilege.) I call this "respecting" our food. Whether you are eating a candy bar or a spinach salad, sit down and make it special.

Tips for take-out

By now you are saying, "This woman is nuts! How can I work all day, then pick up kids and get them to music lessons, Scouts, soccer practice . . . and feed them in between?"

Hold on! You can do it. There are many ways to make those rushed meals healthier and a little more relaxed. Try going into the fast food restaurant and sitting down to eat for just ten to fifteen minutes. If you're getting home delivery, call in the order before you leave work, timing it so the food will get there right after you arrive home—sit down and eat for a few minutes before rushing off to activities.

If you have to go straight from work to pick up the kids from daycare or school and then to an activity, bring snacks with you—bags of nuts and raisins, or crackers and string cheese and pieces of fruit. After the activity, go out for a quick meal, order in, or make a fast dinner at home—just sit down together and enjoy whatever you are eating.

In the next chapter, we'll talk about how to make a fast food meal more nutritious.

Eat together as a family

Okay, your kids are sitting at the table—are you eating with them?

It's tempting to feed young kids before eating ourselves. A peaceful meal is inviting! But think about it: how can our children learn to eat properly if they are not eating with their parents? We can *tell* our child to chew with his mouth closed, take smaller bites, use his napkin, say please and thank you; but by *showing* him these things, he will be much more likely to learn them and do them.

If you like to eat dinner later, give kids a snack around four or five PM and then have dinner together at seven or eight. Family meals can be some of our richest parenting times. Not only do we model and teach table manners, we also model and teach our kids how to enjoy group conversations. (And of course when they have trouble settling down, there's always that three-strike rule!)

Granted, there are times when a schedule is just so busy that sitting down for family meals is impossible. Have you noticed that sports practices for elementary-school kids usually take place during the dinner hour? What to do? One solution is to wait and have dinner as a family at seven-thirty or eight PM. On practice days, make an easy dinner—maybe a crockpot meal or leftovers that can be heated up quickly (you'll find some quick and easy recipes in chapter 13).

One family I know was never together at dinnertime, so they had breakfast together every day. (Both parents had jobs that required frequent evening meetings, but they still wanted to eat together.) They managed to have their teenagers get up early enough to sit down with them for breakfast—even though it was at six AM and they were a bit sleepy at times.

Anything is possible. I did not say it was easy! It's okay to be creative and find something that works for you. If daily family meals can't happen, try finding a couple of days in the week when you eat one meal—any meal—together. It will be an especially important goal to set as your kids enter middle and high school.

"This all sounds fine and dandy," you might say, "but my experiences of family meals have been disasters!" We can't deny that our childhood memories influence us as parents today.

I was recently co-teaching a weight management class with a mental health therapist, Laurie Koski, MSW. My job was to present the nutritional information, which included the benefits of family meals. Laurie's job was to talk about emotions around eating.

She asked folks about their experiences at the dinner table when they were kids. Some were horrific—silent, uncomfortable meals where no one said anything for fear of angering a parent . . . abusive conversation from an alcoholic parent . . . a requirement to sit in front of a food until it was eaten . . . explosive anger when someone spilled her milk . . . dirty looks from a mother who thought her daughter was overeating . . . and questions like "Do you really want that much?" or "Should you be eating that second helping of potatoes?"

> Feeling gratitude and not expressing it is like wrapping a present and not giving it.
> —William Arthur Ward

These experiences resulted in many of these folks developing very dysfunctional eating habits. They certainly did not think of family meals as warm, enjoyable ways to promote family togetherness. Food and eating conjures up many emotions—according to Laurie, "Food is never neutral." Many of us need to work through our own food issues in order to help our children develop healthy eating habits and a healthy enjoyment of food.

If you find yourself having a difficult time envisioning regular family meals with your kids, think back to your childhood and try to figure out what you might be carrying over from your own negative experiences. Then think about small steps that you could take to promote positive mealtime experiences for yourself and your kids.

Benefits beyond nutrition

Once my children got jobs as teens, getting them home for dinner at the same time was hard, and we had to be flexible to eat together even a few nights each week. We did not have a set dinnertime—it varied depending on our schedules. When at all possible, we ate together as a family. My kids both have fond memories of those dinners. Our conversations would travel from what happened at school to some current event in the news to how to solve some math puzzle—and to discussions about sex, drugs, and alcohol as the kids got older.

Those conversations made us closer as a family, and we still have great family mealtimes whenever either or both of them are home.

Think about ways you can increase the number of times per week that your family eats together. It is well worth the trouble! Research shows that kids who eat family meals at least five times per week are less apt to be overweight than those who rarely eat family meals. Other studies show a lower incidence of high-risk behaviors (early sex, drug/alcohol abuse, and smoking) in kids who have regular family meals.

This doesn't mean that kids who eat family meals will be perfect by any means—I can attest to that! But family meals definitely promote communication between parents and children, which is worth a lot.

Involve your kids in shopping, cooking, and cleanup

We have about eighteen years to teach our kids how to be adults. That includes teaching them how to feed themselves—from buying the food to storing it, preparing it, and cleaning it up.

When my kids were toddlers and preschoolers, I relished being able to go to the grocery store occasionally without them. Of course, taking just one was much easier than both. When they were with me, I'd talk to them about what I was putting in our cart: "We're not buying peaches because they are out of season and too expensive . . . we're buying a certain type of apple, because they are nice and ripe and a better price than another type," I'd explain. By the time they were nine or ten, old enough to help with the shopping, they knew quite a bit about what to buy and what to leave on the shelf—for both nutritional and economic considerations.

I could send them to different parts of the store to find things on my list and give them parameters for how to choose the right food: cereal needed to have at least three grams of fiber and less than seven grams of sugar (one-and-a-half teaspoons) per serving; bread needed to be 100 percent whole grain; apples needed to be firm, with no bruises; oranges needed to feel heavy and have fairly smooth skin.

The really positive thing about involving them in the shopping when they were young was that once they got their driver's licenses, I could have them help me make a list, give them money, and send them to the grocery store without me. (Kids will do anything to get driving privileges!) I knew that sending them to the store would result in a few more "treats" coming home than I would have bought—I figured that was the price of not going shopping myself.

Encourage young cooks

From the time kids are very young they can help with making meals at home. A two-year-old can help tear lettuce for salad. A preschooler can pour ingredients into a bowl of whatever you are whipping up. A five-year-old can stir something on the stove with some close supervision, and an eight-year-old can make scrambled eggs.

Kids need to be in the kitchen, helping to prepare meals, so that they will learn to cook and be contributing members of the family. This helps them to appreciate the food that is served and certainly helps them to be more willing to try new things. This will pay huge dividends to you—by the time they are in fifth or sixth grade, they can be responsible for preparing some simple family meals by themselves.

My children both were totally responsible for preparing one dinner per week in the summer, by the time they were eleven and thirteen years old. They decided what they wanted to make and made a list of what they needed. The rules were that they had to make something from scratch. We ended up with some pretty nice meals! Nothing is better than coming home from work to a meal that someone else has prepared.

Cleanup is also important—putting food away so that it won't spoil, washing pots and pans, and loading/unloading the dishwasher are necessary parts of life. When kids are two or three years old, they love to help you clean up the kitchen—somehow, by eight or nine the shine has worn off those clean-up tasks. But why should mom or dad be the ones to do all the dirty work?

Working together with one of my kids to clean the kitchen resulted in lots of great conversation. We just naturally talked with each other and it made cleaning up more enjoyable than it would have been for either of us alone.

Actions for the week
choose one or two that you are not already doing

1. Think about your family's lifestyle—how much time do you spend eating while watching TV? Where do you and your children eat most often? How can you start to change this to eating at the table without the TV on, even if it's one meal a week?

2. How often, and where, does your family eat out? If it's fast food, try and sit down at a table for at least one of the meals.

3. Think about ways you can get your kids involved in preparing meals.

4. We are all at different places in our eating styles—you may well be doing all of the things discussed in this chapter. But if you see room for improvement, pick one thing you want to work on and go for it. Don't worry if it takes several weeks to make it a habit.

5. Pause before eating to give thanks for your meal.

The "Whats" of Eating

T HE DAY STARTED OUT BADLY—YOU OVERSLEPT. Your son
needs cash for a field trip; your daughter needs to bring her
science project to school and it's too fragile to carry on the
bus . . . you haven't hit the grocery store this week, so there's
"nothing good to eat" for breakfast (according to your kids). Being the
resourceful parent you are, you give the kids and yourself cheese and
crackers and raisins for breakfast (at least you have enough of that)
and send some dried fruit and nut trail mix for morning snacks. You've
prepaid for lunches at school, so no worries about making lunch.

You search through pockets of coats and pants to find enough cash
for the field trip, drive the kids to school with the science project, and get
yourself to work. This is not the kind of morning you want to repeat, but
everyone arrived where they needed to be and had a balanced breakfast to
boot (cheese gives protein, raisins are a fruit, and crackers are made from
grain). Whew!

● ● ● ● ● ● ● ● ● ● ● ● ●

While many of us might hold to the old paradigm of a "hot" breakfast as
the ideal (you know: eggs, bacon, toast, and perhaps that large glass of fresh-
squeezed orange juice), there are actually many food combinations that
provide nutritious and balanced meals—like the cheese, raisins, and crackers
in the story above.

So, what *should* we feed our kids to help them grow up to be healthy? And
how do we get them to *eat* those healthy foods—especially with our rushed
lives?

What does a healthy balanced diet look like?

We've all seen the "food pyramid"—it was altered a few years ago to focus more on whole grains and vegetables. This message is even stronger with the My Plate campaign, introduced in 2011. You can get lots of details at www.choosemyplate.gov.

The federal government's recommendations, from "My Plate" are the following.

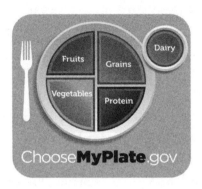

My Plate

Grains 1 serving =	*Vegetables* 1 serving =	*Fruits* 1 serving =	*Milk/Dairy* 1 serving =	*Meat/Beans* 1 serving =
1 oz. slice bread 4" pancake 6" tortilla 1 small muffin ½ cup cooked cereal, pasta, or rice 1 cup ready-to-eat cereal	½ cup cooked vegetables 6 baby carrots ½ sweet potato ½ large tomato 1 cup raw, leafy greens 4 oz. vegetable juice	1 cup sliced fruit 32 grapes 8 large strawberries 1 medium whole fruit ¼ cup dried fruit	8 oz. milk 8 oz. yogurt 1½ oz. cheese ⅓ cup shredded cheese 2 cups cottage cheese	¼ cooked beef patty or chicken breast (1 oz.) 1 egg 1 oz. cheese ¼ cup cooked beans 12 almonds 1 Tbsp. peanut butter
Toddlers: 3–4/day 4–6 yrs: 4–5/day 7–10 yrs: 5–8/day Teens: 8–10/day	Toddlers: 3/day 4–6 yrs: 3–5/day 7–10 yrs: 5+/day Teens: 5+/day	Toddlers: 1/day 4–6 yrs: 1½/day 7–10 yrs: 2/day Teens: 2+/day	Toddlers: 2/day 4–6 yrs: 2–3/day 7–10 yrs: 3/day Teens: 3/day	Toddlers: 2–3/day 4–6 yrs: 2–4/day 4–10 yrs: 4–5/day Teens: 5–7/day

What about fats and sweets—aren't those bad for us?

We get fats in nuts, peanut butter, avocados, oils used in cooking and in salad dressings, butter, margarine, cheese, ice cream, one percent or higher milk, meat, and mayonnaise used on breads, as well as from many snack foods and processed foods. Some fats are essential to our health; oils that are liquid at room temperature provide more of the "essential fatty acids" we need than do solid fats (butter, margarine, shortening, and the fat in meats and dairy products).

If your child is overweight or gaining weight faster than she should, you want to keep fats on the moderate side. Use nonfat or one-percent milk,

The Scoop on Sugar

n our frenzy to cut fat from our diets, we have added much more sugar. Researchers are now telling us that a diet high in sugar is just as detrimental as a diet high in saturated or trans fats. The sugars added to foods include the much maligned high fructose corn syrup, sucrose (table sugar), and honey. Each of these is approximately 50 percent glucose and 50 percent fructose.

We have been hearing about lots of evils associated with fructose—and they are true—when eaten in excess: it gives you extra calories, and it tends to be metabolized in a way that raises triglycerides and cholesterol. It is thought to increase hormones that make you hungry and block the action of the hormone leptin that makes you feel full. Fructose is also implicated in insulin resistance, the main cause of type 2 diabetes. The fructose part of sugar may be what makes people feel as if they are addicted to sugar. These negative effects of fructose can be decreased by exercise and a high fiber intake, which brings us to the sugar that occurs naturally in foods.

The sugar in fruit and sweet vegetables (for example, yams, sweet potatoes, peas, and carrots) is what makes them sweet; when we eat fruits and vegetables we get lots of vitamins and minerals, fiber, and sugar. The sugar in fruits and vegetables is a combination of glucose, fructose, and sucrose (the same as the sugar that we add to foods in the forms of high fructose corn syrup, honey, or table sugar).

avoid deep-fried foods, and go easy on the butter, mayonnaise, and other added fats. It is important to include some healthy fats such as nuts, avocado, peanut butter, and canola, safflower, or olive oil to help make foods taste good, provide essential fatty acids, and help her to feel full and satisfied after a meal.

If your child is underweight, you want to increase those "healthy" fats, so that you can increase calories without increasing the total amount of food he needs to increase his weight. Regardless of his weight, you do not want to give him a lot of "saturated fats"—solid fats, like those you find in meats, butter, and cheese. These are the type of fats that can increase blood cholesterol levels and eventually increase risk for heart disease. This is especially important if parents have high cholesterol levels, or if there are family members who have heart disease or have had heart attacks or strokes at a young age (under sixty to seventy years old).

Sugar is a "simple" carbohydrate. It is not "bad" in and of itself—the problem is that we eat too much added sugar. Over the past century our intake of added sugar has increased by about 500 percent; it has doubled over the past thirty years. That has resulted in a huge increase in calories that do not give us much nutritional benefit.

When we eat candy or drink soda pop or even fruit juice, we get sugar and not much else. We definitely do not get the fiber that helps decrease the negative effects of fructose. All of us benefit from keeping sweets and added sugars on the low side, but totally restricting sweets will just make our kids seek them out when we are not looking. When we make sure that our meals include plenty of high fiber, whole grains, vegetables, and fruits to fill our kids up on complex carbohydrates, we can satisfy them with small desserts or treats that give a little sugar but are not excessive (see the dessert section in chapter 13).

> One should eat to live,
> not live to eat.
> —Benjamin Franklin,
> *quoting Socrates*

Parents need to compromise at times: When my friend's kids were young, she didn't buy highly sugared cereal on a regular basis. She did buy it, though, for camping trips, and she let each kid choose one box of sugary cereal

Sample Menus

	Toddlers	4–6 yrs	7–10 yrs	Teens
Breakfast	¼–½ cup oatmeal cooked with 1 Tbsp. finely ground nuts	½ cup oatmeal cooked with 2 Tbsp. chopped nuts	¾–1 cup oatmeal cooked with 2–4 Tbsp. chopped nuts	1–2 cups oatmeal cooked with 4–6 Tbsp. chopped nuts
	¼ orange	½ orange	1 orange	1 slice whole grain toast with peanut butter
	8 oz. milk	8 oz. milk	8 oz. milk	1 orange
				8 oz. milk
Snack	½ oz. string cheese	1 oz. string cheese	1 apple	1 apple
	¼ apple	½ apple	1 oz. whole grain pretzels	1 oz. whole grain pretzels
Lunch	½ peanut butter sandwich	½–¾ peanut butter sandwich	1 turkey sandwich	1 turkey sandwich
	¼–½ cup cooked and chilled broccoli spears dipped in Ranch-style dressing	½ cup raw sliced broccoli and cauliflower with Ranch-style dressing	½–1 cup raw broccoli and cauliflower with Ranch-style dressing	1 string cheese
	4 oz. milk	16 grapes	16–32 grapes	1 cup raw broccoli and cauliflower with Ranch-style dressing
		4 oz. milk	8 oz. milk	32 grapes
				8 oz. milk
Snack	1 graham cracker square	2 graham cracker squares	1 slice toast with 1 Tbsp. peanut butter	2 slices toast with peanut butter
	6 cooked, chilled baby carrots	6 baby carrots	6–12 baby carrots	12 baby carrots
Dinner	2 oz. baked chicken (drumstick)	2–3 oz. baked chicken (thigh)	3–4 oz. baked chicken (large thigh or small ½ breast)	3–6 oz. baked chicken (small thigh and small ½ breast)
	⅛–¼ medium baked yam with ½ tsp. butter	¼–½ medium baked yam with 1 tsp. butter	½ medium yam with 1 tsp. butter	1 medium yam with 1–2 tsp. butter
	¼–½ cup green beans sautéed in olive oil and garlic	½ cup green beans sautéed in olive oil and garlic	¾ cup green beans sautéed in olive oil and garlic	1 cup green beans sautéed in olive oil and garlic
	½ canned or fresh peach	½–1 canned or fresh peach	1 canned or fresh peach	1 whole grain roll
	4 oz. milk	8 oz. milk	8 oz. milk	1 canned or fresh peach
				8 oz. milk
Snack	½–1 slice whole grain toast with butter	1 slice whole grain toast with butter	1 slice whole grain toast with butter	1 slice whole grain toast with butter

on their birthdays. She compromised on her day-to-day cereals by buying ones that contained whole grains and some added sugar, but sugar was not the first ingredient (these were used as toppings for very low-sugar cereals).

When those high-sugar birthday cereals were in the house, she didn't consider them "breakfast"—they were an extra or a snack food. A bowl of sugared cereal and milk did not cut it for breakfast! There needed to be something more substantial with it if the kids were going to make it through the morning (such as toast with peanut butter, or an egg).

How is it possible to eat all the food that's recommended?

Okay, so the sample menu in the accompanying chart is an example of how to meet daily nutritional needs—but let's be realistic! How does a busy family fit this all in?

To start, food preparation needs to be convenient, especially for single parents and families with two working parents. We want our kids to do those "extras," like music lessons, Scouts, and sports—and unfortunately, in our busy society, these things usually happen after parents' work hours, which is during the traditional dinner hour.

That means you might need to eat really fast dinners a few nights of the week. (Oftentimes, we tend to consider "fast food" as "junk food"—but it doesn't have to be!)

Some easy ways to "jazz up" fast food, yet still keep it nutritious

Try going to a fast-food restaurant and ordering burgers with side salads and milk to drink; if you order fries, get one large order for the whole family. Go in and sit down to eat, or take it home and eat it at the table.

Order pizza on whole wheat crust or get take-out chicken teriyaki (with brown rice, if available) on your way home from work, and serve sliced oranges and prewashed green salad or baby carrots with the pizza or teriyaki at home.

Make super-fast dinners at home (and save some money)

Buy a jar of spaghetti sauce (look for the variety lowest in sodium), sauté boneless, skinless chicken in a little olive oil, and pour the sauce over it. While the chicken is sautéing, boil the water and cook some whole grain pasta and, voila! You have a pretty healthy entrée.

Add a spinach orange salad (made with prewashed spinach and a can of mandarin oranges from the grocery store) or some frozen vegetables heated in the microwave or on top of the stove and you have an extremely healthy meal, made in less than one-half hour. To be even faster, just add raw or frozen spinach or other vegetables to the spaghetti sauce and you have a meal in one dish.

Or you might sauté some ground turkey, chicken, or extra-lean beef in a little olive oil, or in a nonstick pan, with garlic powder, onion powder, chili powder, and cumin. Add a can of drained and rinsed black, pinto, or kidney beans and ¼ to ½ cup water and allow the mixture to simmer until you are ready to eat. Have your kids grate some cheese (or buy it already grated); tear up some romaine or green leaf lettuce; chop a tomato; and heat some whole grain flour or corn tortillas in the microwave. You have a delicious taco dinner in about fifteen minutes.

When time is really limited, serve peanut butter and jam sandwiches, fruit, baby carrots, and milk; cereal, milk, and fruit; or whole grain toaster waffles topped with berries and yogurt for dinner. There is nothing magic about the foods we typically eat for breakfast, lunch, and dinner. When I was a teenager, I ate cold dinner leftovers for breakfast on a regular basis (that was before microwaves!).

Super-fast breakfasts

What about breakfast—we don't have time to "cook" a nourishing breakfast every morning! We want our kids to have a balance of protein, carbohydrate, and fat to fill them up and give them the energy and brainpower to concentrate at school, as well as to get some vitamins and minerals into them.

Here are some quick and easy ideas:

- Whole grain, ready-to-eat cereal (for example, Cheerios, shredded wheat, bran flakes, Wheat Chex) topped with milk, nuts and fruit, and a little sugar, honey, or a couple of tablespoons of sugared cereal (if you want to add more "sweetness" than that in the fruit). This is everything your child needs in one bowl—whole grain for energy, fiber, and B vitamins and a little protein; milk for calcium and protein; fruit for more fiber and vitamins and antioxidants; nuts for healthy fat, vitamin E, more protein, and fiber. Make a cup of cocoa with milk and chocolate powder heated in the microwave or on top of the stove (this gives far more protein and calcium than do the instant hot chocolate mixes that are mixed with water).
- Toasted whole wheat English muffin or bread, peanut or almond butter and jam, a piece of fruit, and a glass of milk or cup of cocoa.
- Leftover pizza and fruit, or any dinner leftovers, heated in the microwave, and fruit or vegetable and a glass of milk.
- Whole wheat or corn tortilla topped with cheese and heated in the oven or microwave; garnish with sliced tomatoes or eat a piece of fruit on the side.
- For a really rushed morning—a sandwich bag of dry, whole grain cereal mixed with nuts and raisins and a string cheese on the way out the door.

Any of these breakfasts will keep your child going for three or four hours and go a long way toward meeting her nutritional needs for the day.

School lunches—"we just don't have time to make them!"

School lunch programs are required to include protein, grain, fruit or vegetable, and milk in each meal. Recent laws passed at both federal and state levels are making these meals healthier than ever before. What worked for my family was having my kids make their lunches on days they didn't like what was on the school menu and on mornings that we were less rushed, and then eat school lunch the rest of the time.

My requirement was that lunch included a grain, a protein, and fruit or vegetable. One day, my daughter put together a sandwich bag of Raisin Bran, some cheese, and an apple—I told her I didn't think that was a very good lunch, but she pointed out that it indeed met my requirements. "Well, okay, but the Raisin Bran is going to turn to crumbs." She stuck to her guns but didn't make that particular lunch again.

Another time, she wanted a prepackaged lunch tray that included processed meat and cheese, crackers, and a juice drink in the worst way. I was not about to buy one—these products were high in salt and fat, had no fiber and little nutritional value other than calories and protein. She persisted in asking, and I finally said she could buy one with her own money. She did—she took it to school for lunch but did not ask for one again.

When our kids entered middle school, we gave them an allowance that covered school supplies, clothes, and school lunches; if they made their lunches at home, they could use that part of the money for themselves. Amazing! They found time to make their lunches several days each week. If nothing else, there was always bread, peanut butter and jam, and fruits and vegetables that they could take.

Healthy goals are to include protein (which includes milk and dairy products as well as meats, poultry, fish, eggs, beans, and nuts), whole grains, and vegetables and/or fruit with each meal and at least one of these with each snack. There are going to be those days when your family's eating is not perfectly balanced, but aiming for these goals will take your family further along the road to healthy eating.

What if your child refuses to eat the food you've prepared?

As the parent, you get to decide what is going to be served for a meal or snack. Your child gets to decide if, what, and how much he is going to eat of that meal or snack.

Most of the time there will be something in a meal that your child likes; his health will not be impaired if he does not eat a little of everything on the table. He may even decide that he is not hungry and does not want to eat anything— that is fine! But he needs to wait until the next planned meal or snack before he eats again—remember the two-to-four hours between meals and snack idea.

If you are offering three meals and two or three snacks each day, your child has enough options for eating that he can easily meet his needs even if he skips a meal.

Exceptions to this recommendation include children who are failing to thrive, have eating disorders, or have chronic illnesses that affect their appetite. In these cases, you want to make sure your child is being followed by a healthcare team that includes a registered dietitian with experience in pediatric nutrition and children with special healthcare needs. Even in

Quick Tips for Making Meals Healthy

- Cook three or four cups of prewashed or frozen spinach with jar of spaghetti sauce to serve over whole grain pasta.

- Add one cup finely chopped fresh or frozen broccoli, cauliflower, carrots, or peas to one to two cups mashed potatoes (homemade or instant).

- Add a handful of nuts to your child's breakfast cereal (any kind of cold cereal or hot cereal) to add some protein and healthy fat, which will hold him until lunch.

- Make hot cereal with milk instead of water to increase the protein and calcium.

- Use quick-cooking brown rice to get the same fiber and vitamins in regular brown rice.

- When cooking regular brown rice or dried beans, make enough for several meals and freeze the extra for quick meals on rushed days.

children such as these, cajoling or forced feeding to get a child to eat are inappropriate.

The last thing you want to do is to make a big deal over your child's refusal of a food or to let your child have something different for his meal when he turns up his nose at your food. It may take several instances of seeing a food on his plate, smelling it, feeling it, and/or taking tiny tastes before he is willing to really eat it.

I remember when I was a young child I was not enthusiastic about Chinese foods—the noodles and bean sprouts in chow mein looked a lot like worms to me, and there was no way I was going to eat that! By the time I was eleven or twelve years old, I loved all types of Chinese foods—it just took time for me to "trust" that they were okay.

Think about those foods that you did not like when you were very young but that ended up being favorites by the time you were an adult. The only way you would come to eat them was to see them, smell them, and taste them frequently and see other people enjoying them.

More about this in chapter 6, "Help for Picky Eaters."

Actions for the week
choose one or two that you are not already doing

1. Add a fruit or a vegetable to each meal.
2. Use brown rice or whole grain pasta in place of white rice or pasta.
3. Allow your kids to buy school lunch *without* your feeling guilty.
4. Buy milk rather than soda pop to drink and side salads rather than fries to eat with your burgers or chicken strips at a fast-food restaurant.

Kids Are Made to Be Active

S EVERAL FAMILIES IN OUR NEIGHBORHOOD have kids between about four and seven years old. I see the children ride their bikes and scooters, play elaborate games, and generally have a great time outside all summer long. In the winter, they slide down their yards on anything that will move on snow, build snowmen . . . I love watching these kids enjoy being very active in unstructured play, outside!

Yes, they scrape their knees, fall off their bikes, and are not always as supervised as some in our neighborhood would like, but they are doing what kids are made to do—playing actively and creatively. By the way, none of these kids are either overweight or underweight!

● ● ● ● ● ● ● ● ● ● ● ● ●

Organized activities and sports for kids are fantastic, but they do not give kids all the activity they need. I have far too many overweight young clients who are athletes but who sit in front of the TV or computer and gain excessive weight during their offseasons. This becomes more of a problem as kids hit middle school and high school—they no longer have "recess" at school, they have a lot of homework after school, and they use the TV and video/computer games for fun.

During their sports seasons, they are active for at least two hours per day, five or six days per week. That drops to forty-five to fifty minutes of physical education (if they even have PE) during the rest of the school year and even less during the summer in the offseason. These kids typically lose a little weight during sports seasons, when they are not only very active, but they have less time to "graze" between meals. Only the most serious of youth athletes actually keep active during their offseasons.

With my own kids, I noticed a distinct decrease in physical activity when they started middle school. During elementary school they had two or three recesses each day; they typically played a pick-up game of basketball, soccer, or football during recess. This served two purposes—it gave them great physical exercise, and it helped them to be ready to learn when they got back to class. They played outside after school as well.

Once in middle school, they had four-minute passing periods between classes and a twenty-five-minute lunch break. The gym was open for basketball, but the gym certainly could not hold all the kids who had the same lunch break . . . and the teachers and administrators wondered why seventh- and eighth-grade boys, especially, had so much trouble sitting still and learning in class.

The children had physical education two out of three trimesters each year, so some of those kids had no physical activity for a third of the school year. After-school sports were a great option and were open to "most" students (those whose grades were low were not allowed to participate). For some reason, kids seem to quit "playing" outside in the neighborhood after school when they are about middle-school age.

We know that just by increasing physical activity of all kids by fifteen to thirty minutes per day, we can seriously decrease the incidence of childhood obesity. This in turn will decrease the number of kids who go on to develop type 2 diabetes—and this will decrease our national healthcare costs tremendously. So . . . what can we do?

Making play fun again

The most powerful thing we can do to get kids more active is to decrease inactivity. National guidelines tell us to limit "screen time" that is not associated with doing homework to less than two hours per day. Two hours is a lot of time for a kid to sit on her behind for entertainment—that does not include time sitting to do homework, read for pleasure, or talk on the phone to friends.

But 26 percent of all kids spend *more than four hours per day* in front of a TV, video game, or computer for entertainment. All this sitting time takes away from time to be active. Any activity will work muscles and burn more energy than sitting in front of a TV or computer.

I recommend allowing kids a certain number of hours per week for screen entertainment—six to eight hours per week allows for an occasional TV show, plus a movie or two on the weekend or a couple of hours playing video games with a friend occasionally. In most cases, with a limit of six to eight hours per week, there would be some days with no screen-time entertainment. If your kids and their friends are playing cards or board games, they are moving a whole lot more than if they are watching TV.

Outside play

Kids do best when they have some unstructured playtime outside each day. Young kids are pretty easy to entertain—they will ride a bike or tricycle up and down the same stretch of sidewalk, swing on a swing set or tire swing, and climb on a jungle gym for a long, long time. Older kids and teenagers are far more apt to figure out something active to do outside if the option of TV or video games is not available. Building forts, digging holes, climbing trees, walking to the store, taking the bus to the local swimming pool, going for a bike ride, playing team games—even hide-and-seek—they'll find plenty of things to do.

As parents, it is very difficult to let our kids be independent, but many of our fears are truly unfounded. Many parents cite kidnapping by strangers as a number one fear—however much the media would have us believe differently, stranger kidnappings are extremely rare! Being hit by a car while bicycle riding or crossing the street is a more rational fear, but there are many things we can do to decrease those risks.

We need to teach our kids safe ways of walking, crossing streets, riding bikes, and using the city bus system, starting from a very young age. If we do this, by the time they are ten or eleven years old they can safely walk or ride their bike to school and cross busy streets, and by the time they are twelve many kids can negotiate the city bus system (if your community has one) to get themselves to activities.

Inside play

Just because the weather is crummy and outside play is not practical, it does not mean that the TV needs to be turned on.

For young kids, keep a costume box or drawer and let your kids dress up and play make-believe.

Bring out the blankets and sheets and let your kids turn the living room into a fort, using furniture and blankets—have a picnic lunch inside their make-believe cave. (Put a washable tablecloth on the floor to protect your carpet!)

Encourage your kids and their friends to play hide-and-seek (be sure to make it clear what areas of the house are off limits).

Encourage older kids to entertain the younger ones in these activities (they will be active and have fun as well, but it won't be "un-cool" since they are "helping" with the young kids).

Have kids build elaborate structures with blocks, Legos, Duplos, Erector sets, and similar construction toys.

Kids love to do art projects—keep construction paper, crayons, glue, and paints around. Give your kids a theme for their artwork such as their favorite story, a holiday or religious observance, or their favorite animal at the zoo. You might even have them cut out foods from old magazines and glue them to a paper plate to show a healthy meal.

Without much trouble you can think of other ways to keep your kids occupied on a rainy day, without ever turning on the TV.

Teach your kids to clean up the mess they make from their inside activities! Have them put the costumes back in the box or drawer, fold up the blankets, put the furniture back in place, and clean up the art projects. So many people would rather let their kids do something neat and easy, like watch TV, because the messes they make doing other more active things are overwhelming. Start having them help clean up as soon as they can walk. It is amazing how well an eighteen-month-old can put toys back in the toy box.

Organized sports activities

Kids benefit greatly from being on teams, provided the coaching is positive and encouraging, but we have to be careful not to push too hard or overschedule our kids. Mine started playing soccer when they were in first grade—it was low-key and fun. Definitely good entertainment for the parents and grandparents! The kids gradually went from "bumble bee soccer"—all running in a pack—to actually playing positions. They learned how to work as a team, how to follow a coach's instructions, *and* they got great physical activity. It was overall a very positive experience.

As the kids and their friends got older, and the sport got more competitive and expensive, many of them dropped out, while some went on to play "select" soccer. The not-so-competitive club team just didn't exist for middle school and above. "Select" and high school soccer were extremely competitive, so very few kids actually had a shot at making those teams. However, school sports such as cross-country running and track tended to be "non-cut" sports where anyone and everyone in the school can join.

Sports like Ultimate (Frisbee), volleyball, and lacrosse have become popular for teenagers—intramural teams are formed, and in many cases kids who would never be on the basketball, baseball, or football team are on these teams. Many kids want to be on a "sports team," but they do not want to put in the time or endure the pressure of more conventional and competitive teams. This is quite reasonable; not everyone is a super athlete, but everyone needs to be active!

> Luck is what happens when preparation meets opportunity.
> —Seneca

Individual activities

All children benefit from learning to swim. Knowing how to swim opens up a great avenue for physical activity, and it increases the safety level of a child who goes to the local swimming pool, attends "swim parties," and has fun doing other water activities. Many cities have indoor and outdoor public swimming pools; open or family swim sessions are great family outings, even in the dead of winter.

Bicycle riding is another amazing activity for kids and adults. Starting on a tricycle or a balance bike (foot-propelled without pedals) as a young preschooler and then advancing to a bicycle is one of those rites of passage for kids. Be sure your children wear helmets when they start on anything with wheels.

When they are ready to learn to ride a two-wheeler, try riding on grass—it truly diminishes the fear of falling. We discovered that by accident when our daughter learned to ride a bike—when she rode onto the grass, she had less fear and so had better balance than on the pavement. After a day of riding on grass, she was up for riding anywhere.

Going on family bike rides is the best way to teach your kids safe riding techniques. Start on low-traffic roads or bike paths and gradually work up to riding on busier streets after your child has mastered safe riding. Teach your kids the importance of wearing a helmet by wearing one yourself!

If you are not comfortable cycling in your community, check out cycling classes—many communities have organizations that offer bicycle safety classes. It will be impossible to feel comfortable cycling with your kids if you are not confident yourself.

Bicycling has amazing payoffs as well—it gives your kids independence. By the time they are in middle school, they can get themselves to many activities on their bikes.

Walking is the best of all "individual" activities! We teach our kids to use their feet as transportation from the time we start walking with them in a stroller or in a baby front or back carrier.

If you are within walking distance of your children's elementary school, walk them to school, whenever possible. If they ride a school bus, walk them to the bus stop.

If you are within walking distance to work (a true luxury!), walk to work. If you can take a bus or train to work, walk to the stop.

For some of us, walking is not a true option, because of lack of sidewalks on busy streets or long distances to school or work or stores. How can we increase our walking?

When we go to the grocery store, park at the far end of the parking lot. When we are doing errands in town, park at a central location and walk from one business to another, especially when we have our kids with us.

Any time our kids see us walking to get where we want to go, they are getting the idea that walking is a good thing (even if they are complaining the whole way). One of the nice things about walking is that it can be a part of our "daily activities" rather than something we are specifically doing to get "exercise."

Walking and hiking are great recreational activities as well. I have the extreme blessing of living in a beautiful place with lots of walking trails; my home is a five-minute walk from the River Trail, a beautiful trail on the Deschutes River maintained by our city parks and recreation department. I enjoy this trail by myself, with friends, with my husband, and with our kids when they come home. What I really love is seeing lots of parents walking or running on the trail with their kids; these families are of all shapes and sizes, not just "super fit" people—which tells me that people really do enjoy being active when given the chance!

Other individual activities are newer on the scene—active-play video games. To that I say, Yes! Fight fire with fire! If we are going to be using video games, why not use video games to get people moving? There are dancing, bowling, skiing, boxing, tennis, and other games. I applaud companies for using this technology to come up with something that is actually healthful. These games can be used by kids and parents together and are a novel way to increase physical activity.

The long and the short of it is that our kids need to be active, and we are our kids' role models for an active lifestyle!

Actions for the week
choose one or two that you are not already doing

1. Set limits on television and video games. Establish a certain number of hours per week and have each child keep a chart of how much time she has spent. Once her hours are used up, the TV and video games are off limits. If she wants to save up her hours for a marathon session, so be it. Just make sure that you have the last word in negotiating how many hours for the week.

2. Go for a walk with your children or with each child individually.

3. Plan some inside activities for the next rainy day.

4. Sign up for a bicycle safety class in your community.

5. Buy yourself and your child bike helmets if you do not already have them.

Part Two

Putting Things in Perspective

Teaching Kids About Healthy Eating

M Y DAUGHTER SUZANNE WAS TWO-AND-A-HALF YEARS old and playing with playdough by herself at the kitchen table while I washed dishes. Her playdough was "chicken," and she was talking to herself, saying over and over again, "I'm cutting all the fat off this chicken, bad fat . . ." I stopped what I was doing and thought—how exactly did she get that message?

I typically cut the skin and fat off chicken and other meat before cooking it, but did I talk about it as I did it? Had I ever told her that "fat was bad"? I wasn't really sure whether this was good or not, but one thing I did realize— kids pick up on what we do and say very early on, and I'd better make sure that I was giving the messages that I wanted my kids to get.

● ● ● ● ● ● ● ● ● ● ● ● ●

Our kids learn their eating habits from us, their parents, more than anyone else. Yes, they learn about nutrition in preschool and school, but what they see and learn at home has the most sticking power!

If they see us eating on the run, skipping meals, grabbing chips and soda pop for our snacks, they will see those habits as normal adult eating.

Three incredibly easy steps to healthy eating
Step 1: Model healthy eating for your children

Chapter 7 talks about healthy adult eating. This is more important than anything else; nothing we say to our kids will override what they see us do. The same goes for any other health message we want to give to our kids—it is difficult for them to believe that smoking is a problem, for example, if they see us smoking; it is difficult for them to see exercise is important if we are physically inactive.

Step 2: Talk to your kids about why you are making different family food choices

Tell them why you buy dried fruit rather than fruit snacks; why you buy whole grain bread rather than white bread; why you don't buy potato chips and cheese puffs very often; why you insist on a piece of fruit and a vegetable in their school lunches; why you use the really small dishes or teacups for ice cream rather than the cereal bowls; why you don't buy apple juice or juice boxes. Our kids see what others are eating and they want to fit in; it can be helpful for them to understand why their lunches or snacks might look different.

When you are at the grocery store, talk to your kids about why you are buying certain products:

Local and in-season fruits and vegetables versus imported or out-of-season. Foods that are local and seasonal can be picked at a riper stage, do not sit in storage for transportation for as long a time, and thus tend to be higher in nutrients.

Oatmeal in a large box or in bulk versus packets of instant oatmeal. Plain oatmeal is a great high-fiber, very low sugar cereal, but the little instant packets have lots of added salt and sugar. You can add apples, cinnamon, and raisins and a little sugar to plain oatmeal and have a much healthier breakfast than if you eat instant apple raisin cinnamon oatmeal. (This is also a great way to give them an economics lesson—the larger boxes or bulk oatmeal costs much less per serving than the instant stuff does.)

Lean meats, chicken, turkey, and fish versus fatty meats such as ribs, prime steaks, bacon, or sausage. The fatty meats have more saturated fat and cholesterol, which are not good for our hearts. The very lean meats give us plenty of protein and iron and vitamins, with far less fat.

We make lots of decisions at the grocery store based on nutritional value. Talking about it helps reinforce the lessons our kids get by watching us eat a healthy diet.

Step 3: Involve your kids in food decisions

At the grocery store, teach your kids how to pick quality fruits and vegetables and how to choose healthy cereals and packaged foods.

Have your kids help to plan meals at home. If you have decided on a specific main dish for dinner, let kids plan the vegetables and/or fruits— green salad, cooked vegetables, cut raw vegetables, fruit salad, plate of sliced fruit, or a combination of any of the above. Let them decide on other side dishes—roasted yams or potatoes, brown rice, whole grain pasta, quinoa, whole-wheat couscous. Let kids plan their school-day breakfasts and lunches. Require some basic healthy parameters such as: a whole grain, a protein, a fruit and/or vegetable, and milk or water (see chapter 13 for breakfast and lunch ideas).

Encourage your kids to participate in all levels of food preparation:

- Gardening—Many kids truly have no idea where their foods come from. Growing at least a few foods at home gives kids a whole new understanding of what it takes to get food on the table. Don't have a yard? Try container gardening for tomatoes, peppers, green beans, and other suitable vegetables.

- Grocery shopping—Allow young children to put produce in bags and take foods off the store shelves and put them in the cart. Give your older kids and teenagers a list and a basket and ask them to find those foods and meet you at a specific location in the store. You will get the grocery shopping done faster and prepare your kids to do it themselves by the time they can drive to the store for you! (Make sure you retain veto power over the items in their carts. You might negotiate with them to choose one treat that is not necessarily "healthy"—just give them a price and size limit).

- Storage—Make sure that you include unloading the car and putting foods away as part of your kids' grocery shopping experience. Teach them to put the newest foods in the back of the refrigerator or cupboards and the older foods in front or on top of the new foods. This will likely require rearranging of the vegetable and fruit drawers of your fridge and shelves in your cupboards, which they might not want to take time to do, but it is part of the process!

- Food preparation—Your kids have helped to plan meals, so now let them do as much preparation as they can. Preschoolers can tear the lettuce for green salad and pour ingredients into a bowl or pan. They can also help by setting and clearing the table. Five- to eight-year-olds can get ingredients out of the cupboards and refrigerator, stir things on the stove with very close supervision, make sandwiches, and load and unload the dishwasher. By the time a child is nine years old, he is capable of cooking simple meals (macaroni and cheese from scratch, spaghetti sauce, scrambled eggs) with supervision while using the stove. By middle-school age, a child can prepare a meal without supervision, as long as they have grown up learning how to use the stove and knives safely.

- Cleanup—No one has truly learned how to cook unless they have learned to clean up. Even if your kids have worked very hard to prepare a meal, they need to be involved in the cleanup (at least cleaning up their cooking mess). Teaching them some clean-as-you-cook techniques can be very useful in the long run.

My mother's claim to fame was that each of her children could put a meal on the table by themselves at nine years of age (she really didn't like cooking, and teaching us to cook was a way for her to do less of it!). Because of that, I developed a love of cooking. I took that idea to heart and made sure that my kids learned to cook, starting at an early age. By the time they were middle-schoolers, I could leave them with instructions on what to make for dinner and have a great meal prepared by the time I walked in the door from work! Even moms who love cooking need a reprieve once in a while.

At the same time that you are teaching your kids meal planning and preparation, you are also giving them nutrition lessons. They will get some nutrition education at school; that will reinforce what you have already taught. In appendix 1 you'll find a breakdown of all the different food groups and why they are important—it's a good place to start educating yourself, if you do not feel that you know enough about nutrition to educate your kids. The references at the end of the book will also give you several ideas for books and websites for improving your knowledge of nutrition with reliable information.

Actions for the week
choose one or two that you are not already doing

1. Ask one of your kids to help plan menus and grocery shop for the week. If you have more than one child, alternate who helps with the planning. Besides being educational, it gives you one-on-one time with each child.

2. Take one of your children to the grocery store with you and talk about what you are buying and why.

3. Give each child a job related to meal preparation at least one day this week—setting the table, making one or more parts of a meal, making lunches, clearing the table, and helping with the dishes.

4. Give your older children a list that includes 25 to 50 percent of what you need to buy at the grocery store. Give them a set amount of time to gather the items and then meet you at a designated place in the store.

Kids' Foods,
or Just a Way to Market Junk?

THE KIDS ARE WATCHING SATURDAY MORNING CARTOONS. About every five minutes they see a commercial for some popular food—toaster pastries, fruit-flavored cereal, juice boxes, yogurt-to-go, fruit snacks, chocolate milk, alphabet soup, macaroni and cheese from a box, cheese-flavored crackers, fast-food "kids' meals." That afternoon they go to the grocery store with their mother. "Pleeease, can't we get _____ ?" Mom sighs and relents—her basket is filling up with just the food she vowed to quit buying. "Mental note to self . . . next week find someone to watch kids while I go grocery shopping."

They pass a fast-food restaurant on the way home. "Mom, we're starving! Pleeease can't we go to the drive-through and get a _____ meal?" It never seems to end.

One mom decided that fast food was not something she was going to cave in on. Every so often she makes her own version of kids' fast-food meals, which she serves in a brown paper sack. The burgers are extra-lean beef or chicken on whole-grain buns, with lettuce and tomatoes; the fries are oven-baked from fresh potato wedges coated with a little oil. She includes a fruit or vegetable. Her kids love these meals—which are likely much tastier and certainly more nutritious (and less expensive) than a fast-food kids' meal. Yes, this is a working mom!

> Our bodies are our gardens, to which our wills are gardeners.
> —William Shakespeare

The television ads aimed at kids may not promote anything so reprehensible as cigarettes and beer, but watch out! The *cereals* advertised contain more sugar than any other single ingredient; one popular kids' brand contains three teaspoons of sugar in a thirty-gram (gm) serving—that is, 41 percent sugar mixed in with some flour, a synthetic vitamin mixture, and artificial colors and flavors. The new "one-third less sugar" version contains almost two-and-a-half teaspoons of sugar in a thirty-two gm serving—that is, 31 percent sugar. Some of these cereals now have a little bit of whole-grain flour and fiber added, but they are far from 100 percent whole grain. And this is supposed to be breakfast?

Juice boxes—even those marked "100 percent juice"—contain mostly apple or grape juice (basically, the sugar water remaining after the fruit pulp is strained out). Fruit sugar is healthy, right? Think harder. White sugar is extracted from sugar cane, a fibrous plant that gives us both molasses—a fairly good source of potassium and iron—and the refined white sugar that we tend to associate with poor nutritional quality.

A traditional *toaster pastry* is about 30 percent sugar with only one-half gm of fiber and very small amounts of any vitamins and minerals.

Healthy Drinks

- When bananas get overripe, peel and put them in a plastic container or bag, or just throw them in the freezer with the peels on—they are excellent vitamin- and potassium-laden smoothie sweeteners.
- Try milk and frozen fruit blended in the blender for a delicious and healthy milk shake.

- One mom in Seattle told me that she had decided to break her kids' reliance on sweet drinks at mealtimes. When her son asked her what there was to drink, she told him "Cascade Kool-Aid"— which of course was water. For folks living in the Northwest part of the United States, the water is fantastic and comes from the Cascade Mountains.

A New Look at Mac 'n' Cheese

f you want to make packaged macaroni and cheese healthier, prepare it according to package instructions; add finely chopped fresh or frozen spinach, broccoli, cauliflower, mixed vegetables, or whatever you have on hand to the macaroni five minutes before it is done cooking. Drain and rinse (to decrease the sodium) a can of water-packed tuna and add that to the finished product—you now have a pretty tasty "tuna noodle casserole" that took less than ten minutes to prepare and includes all the ingredients of a healthy meal.

Other additions all increase protein and nutrients: eggs (add whipped eggs when you mix the cheese sauce into the macaroni— keep the heat on under the macaroni, cheese sauce, and egg mixture until it is boiling, to make sure that the eggs are thoroughly cooked); tofu; beans (garbanzo, black, pinto, red); any leftover meat from a previous meal.

What about typical *boxed or frozen macaroni and cheese* entrees? All are very high in sodium, anywhere from 600 milligrams (mg) of sodium per serving (an option touted as "healthy") to 1470 mg of sodium per serving—that is, from more than one-fourth to almost two-thirds of an adult's total daily recommended sodium intake of 2300 mg per day. Homemade macaroni and cheese can contain as little as 425 mg of sodium per two-cup serving, which is not low-salt but a lot lower than the processed products that are available (you'll find the recipe in chapter 13).

Suffice it to say that our kids are bombarded continually with ads for less-than-healthy foods and beverages. When children watch general programming (not specifically intended just for kids), they see media messages promoting even more unhealthy foods: soda pop, beer, snack foods, and fast foods very high in fat and salt. Unless you are sitting there with them, telling them why the ads are silly or bad, they will truly think they should be eating all these foods.

Let's review some foods and come up with *better alternatives*—after all, eating does not need to be a pleasureless pursuit. Food is an important part of our cultural fabric and we ought to enjoy it. Why else would God have provided such bounty?

Sugared cereals — Try using a couple of tablespoons of one of these cereals or granola on top of a bowl of unsweetened cereal (for instance, plain original Cheerios, shredded wheat, bran flakes). Add some fresh or frozen

Quick Soup Tips

- Brown one-half pound lean ground beef, chicken, turkey, or pork in a saucepan, then drain off fat. Add one ten-ounce can of vegetable, chicken noodle, or other condensed broth-based soup, one can of water, and one cup of frozen mixed vegetables. Cook on medium heat until vegetables are hot, and you have a very simple, nutritious, and tasty vegetable and meat soup that will serve four people. The addition of the very low sodium vegetables and meat stretches the soup to feed more people, so there is less sodium in each serving.

- Prepare any broth-based soup according to label instructions, then add one-fourth cup of diced tofu per person—you have just increased the protein and calcium in the soup.

- Whip up one egg per person and drizzle into any broth-based soup to make an "egg flower" (or "egg drop") type of soup; make sure that the eggs have solidified before serving.

- Add one cup prewashed raw spinach to prepared tomato soup and simmer for two to three minutes until tender; further increase flavor by adding fresh or dried basil, cilantro, or oregano.

- You get the point! You can take something that is not optimally nutritious and increase vitamins, minerals, and protein without spending much time in the kitchen. These are great, fast, and inexpensive ways to feed you and your kids a healthy meal (far healthier and cheaper than a fast food meal).

blueberries, sliced banana, peaches, strawberries . . . and some chopped or ground almonds or walnuts (grind nuts in a coffee grinder for kids under two or three years old, to prevent choking).

Toaster pastries — There are many other options that are quick and easy! A slice of whole-grain toast with butter and jam is a far more nutritious option. If your child must have a toaster pastry, make sure she also is eating some protein (cheese, peanut butter, leftover meat, eggs) and fruit as well. I know my bias is definitely coming out here! Check out the options in chapter 2 for super-fast breakfasts.

Juice boxes — When you want a sweet drink, try chopping some fresh fruit and putting it in the blender; it will become a thick "juice" in a matter of seconds. Add some ice or frozen berries or frozen banana and you have a nutrient-packed smoothie that is balanced in sugar and nutrients. Or go for flavored milk; it still has added sugar, but it also contains protein, calcium, vitamin D, vitamin A, and riboflavin. You will get more nutrition and fewer calories if you add a flavored powder to one-percent or nonfat milk, rather than buying premade flavored milk.

A cup of hot cocoa, made with milk and chocolate powder, is a great way to add extra nutrition to your child's breakfast or after-dinner snack.

Water is the best option for quenching thirst. We are extremely fortunate to have clean, safe drinking water right out of our taps. All of us would do well to make it our first choice.

Packaged macaroni and cheese — You can whip up a pretty good batch of macaroni and cheese by following the recipe in chapter 13; it might take a couple of extra minutes to grate the cheese, but not a lot longer than putting together a boxed version. You can make any macaroni and cheese healthier by adding vegetables and/or meat, poultry, fish, beans, eggs, egg whites, or tofu.

Yogurts-to-go — The biggest problem with these portable snacks is that they promote eating on the run, which is definitely counter to teaching our kids the importance of sitting down and enjoying their food. Flavored yogurts contain a lot of added sugar, which increases calories significantly. A six-ounce carton of flavored yogurt contains a little over three teaspoons of *added* sugar—fifty calories with no nutritional value (this is in addition to the natural milk sugar, lactose).

You can come out way ahead nutritionally by adding fresh or frozen fruit and a teaspoon of honey to six ounces of plain yogurt. Honey has a higher "sweetness factor" than sugar, so between that and the fruit, your yogurt will be plenty sweet. You can also mix plain yogurt with flavored yogurt in a one-to-one ratio and still have a fairly sweet product and only twenty calories from added sugar. (Children under one year of age should not be given honey, due to the risk of botulism—honey contains botulism spores, which don't hurt older children and adults but can build up and release the botulism toxin in the immature guts of infants, causing life-threatening disease.)

Canned soups — These prepared soups can be nutritious, except that it is difficult to find any that are not loaded with sodium. You can make some flavorful, very low sodium soups (see chapter 13 for recipes), but is that realistic given your schedule? If you do make soup, make enough for a few meals and freeze the leftovers in meal-sized containers. If you are buying prepared soups, you can improve the nutritional value and lower the sodium by adding unsalted cooked fresh or frozen vegetables, meat, chicken, tofu, or eggs.

Actions for the week
choose one or two that you are not already doing

1. Talk to your kids about the problems with the foods that are advertised on TV.
2. Give your kids some guidelines for buying cereals—less than five grams of sugar per hundred calories and at least three grams of fiber per hundred calories. Tell them that they can have any cereal they can find that meets those criteria (they won't end up with "cocoa" anything!).
3. Make a quick and easy recipe from chapter 13 rather than using a packaged mix.
4. Use one of the suggestions above to improve the nutritional value of a packaged or canned entree (for example, macaroni and cheese, canned soup).

Help for Picky Eaters

I 'VE HEARD IT ALL: "My daughter will not touch any vegetables." "My son refuses all meats." "I can't get her to drink milk." "He ate everything when he was a baby, but he gets pickier and pickier as he gets older." "She loves vegetables but won't touch fruit." "He eats fruit, but not much else."

● ● ● ● ● ● ● ● ● ● ● ● ● ●

These parents are right—their kids are *very picky* eaters, and for some their pickiness seems to affect growth. What parent wouldn't be concerned!

Parenting brings with it more challenges than it can seem humanly possible to face at times. Nurturing a child's body *and* soul require wisdom, patience, and often a large dose of humor! To start, let's separate some facts from myths in the realm of childhood nutrition.

> Gratitude is when memory is stored in the heart and not in the mind.
>
> —Lionel Hampton

Facts and myths

- "If my child is a light eater, I should just give him free access to food throughout the day."

Myth Children who are underweight and poor eaters who are allowed to graze eat 10 to 25 percent fewer calories than children who have structured meals and snacks. Later, these poor eating habits may lead to obesity.

- "The only way to get my child to eat is to give her meals in front of the television."

  Myth This may seem to work for the short term but does not promote long-term healthy eating habits. Sitting at the table with you and/or other family members for all meals and snacks is the best way for your child to develop healthful eating habits.

- "Children tend to eat better when they are at daycare or preschool."

  Fact Eating in groups often promotes improved intake. If Suzy sees Johnny and Bobby and Mary eating whatever is offered, she is more likely to eat it too. Also, being offered food without someone hovering and telling her to eat one more bite makes meals more enjoyable.

- "Family meals promote healthy eating habits."

  Fact Eating as a family in a positive atmosphere (no TV or other distractions), sitting together at a table, or even on the floor, is a way to model healthy eating. Your young child idolizes you! She wants to be like you! Seeing you eat your meals and enjoy them will eventually pay off (not necessarily today or tomorrow, but in the long run).

  When we make a meal for our family, it tends to be far more balanced than what we make for just one person. When your child participates in regular family meals, he is most likely exposed to a larger variety of foods than when you feed him by himself.

Common sense says that picky eaters will never have a weight problem. Wrong! Many children who were underweight as infants or toddlers become overweight later in childhood or in adulthood.

Many of the ways that we cajole our finicky kids to eat promote obesity as they get older but do not really do much good while they are young and underweight. If your child is both underweight and not growing in height, she may need some special help to increase calorie and nutritional intake; however, all of the recommendations below are still extremely important.

There are also children who are growing just fine, or may even be overweight, who are picky eaters. Regardless of growth rate, we need to promote lifelong healthy eating habits.

What to do when your child seems to "live on air"

First and foremost, make sure your child is getting regular well-child checkups and being weighed and measured.

- Is she following her growth curve?
- Is her weight in good proportion to her length or height?
- If you answered "yes" to the above questions, go to the next section "Assuming your child is growing well." Otherwise, ask yourself:
- Is your child's weight low relative to her length or height?
- Are her weight and/or length falling on the growth curve?

If you answered "yes" to either of the questions above, your child's physician needs to rule out health problems that could cause poor growth.

It may be very helpful for you to see a registered dietitian who has *experience with children.* You can contact the American Dietetic Association (www.eatright.org) or your local medical center to find an appropriate person.

Assuming your child is growing well

Offer meals and snacks no less than two hours and no more than four hours apart.

Do not provide anything other than water between meals and snacks (no juice, diluted juice, milk, and so on), even if he asks for it!

Make sure water is available, but do not let your child carry a water bottle with her—many kids fill their tummies with plain water and then do not want to eat.

Kids need to learn to identify feelings of hunger and fullness. Many parents tell me that if their picky eater asks for something right after a meal, they feel that they have to give it to him, especially if he did not eat anything at the meal. I totally understand the feeling that "my child has to eat something," but no child is going to starve in two hours!

It will take a while to accustom your child to a routine of structured meals and snacks. There will likely be tantrums and crying along the way. Do not start trying to make these changes until you and *all of the people who care for your child* are ready to be consistent—an on-and-off approach to making behavioral changes can cause more harm than good. All the people who are involved with caring for a child need to be on board with the structured meal and snack plan. Grandma can still offer sweets, but your child needs to be sitting at the table at a regular meal or snack time.

Don't cajole, plead, or beg your child to "try one bite" or have a celebration when she does eat a bite. This can be hard to do. Enjoy your meal (easier said than done) and "chill" about whether or not your child eats. Talk about the day, what's going on in the lives of people at the table, anything other than whether your child is eating or not.

Put very small amounts of food on your child's plate; large amounts of food tend to be overwhelming. Better to have your child ask for second and third servings than to have her refuse to eat at all.

Use colorful plates and easy-to-use kids' eating utensils (spoons and forks with broader handles are easier for toddlers and preschoolers to negotiate).

If you are expecting your child to eat in a structured manner, you shouldn't graze your way through the day, either. Give up the habit of eating while driving, doing housework, reading the newspaper, or doing the crossword puzzle. It's important that you lead the way in developing healthy eating habits for your child by modeling them yourself. Remember—our kids are much more likely to do what we do than what we say.

If your child is *not* growing well

The same guidelines apply. You will not do anything good for your child by allowing him to graze all day.

You may need to increase calories by using special milk or adding calorie supplements to foods.

Your child may have one of the many conditions that make it hard for him to get enough nutrition by mouth; some children with special healthcare needs even require tube feeding to supplement eating by mouth. But the same guidelines for eating by mouth apply—in the best of all scenarios, a tube-fed child is given a meal or snack, followed by a tube feeding to make up for the calories he did not eat. Tube fed children require very close follow-up by a registered dietitian with experience in both pediatrics and tube feeding.

Whether your child is a picky eater or not, developing eating patterns is what will help her to know when she is hungry and when she is full. Maintaining appropriate space between meals and snacks is the most important part of getting to that point.

The "short-order cook" trap

Your child is sitting at the table for meals and snacks, and you've got the two-to-four-hour thing down. But she still refuses most of what you offer; you end up making special meals for her so that she will eat *something*.

Excellent—you are off to a good start. But it is okay to quit being a short-order cook! Everyone else who cares for your child needs to know this.

Make sure the meals and snacks that you are making for yourself and your family include at least *one* thing that your picky child likes.

Put a *little* of everything on your child's plate. If he turns up his nose at something, tell him that he does not have to eat it, but it stays on the plate.

Here it comes...screaming "I don't want that on my plate!!!" and throwing the plate on the floor. Strike one. (Remember the "three strikes and you're out" rule from chapter 1?) Make sure he knows he is treading on shaky ground and put food back on his plate (let the dog eat what is on the floor but put a new teaspoon of whatever it was back on the plate).

You may occasionally get all the way to strike three and need to remove him from the table and send him to the other room to play until the family is done with dinner.

Most kids do not like having to play by themselves when everyone else is together. They will *not* get to strike three unless they are truly not hungry, or they are very tired and the meal is a lost cause anyway.

Two hours later, offer him a snack (not dessert!). Good snacks in cases like this include cheese and crackers, one-half or one-fourth of a peanut butter sandwich, yogurt and fruit, or unsweetened cereal and milk.

Remember, hang in there—changing the way you interact with your kids is not for the faint of heart! It is *not* going to be easy. Consistency, consistency, consistency . . . is key.

Now you've put a little of everything on your child's plate, she is being an angel at the dinner table, but she only eats the bread and drinks her milk and asks for more of those. Try your hardest not to get into the "If you take one bite of your broccoli, you can have more bread or milk" pitfall. When we give the impression that the food we want her to try is a less than desirable choice, we reinforce her not wanting it. Let her have as much as she wants of whatever you are serving. For some kids, it does help to not pour the milk until midway into the meal, but other than that I would not put restrictions of how much of any one food she eats.

If you are serving dessert, keep the portions small and serve only enough for one serving per person. Do not deny dessert if your child did not eat dinner (unless of course she has left the table before you serve dessert)—that reinforces the idea of "good foods versus bad foods." Try some healthy desserts—fruit such as watermelon, cantaloupe, sliced peaches, strawberries, applesauce with cinnamon, baked apples or pears with just a dollop of ice cream or vanilla yogurt . . . chocolate pudding, frozen yogurt, sorbet.

Occasionally, more decadent desserts like ice cream sundaes or cake, cookies, pastries, or pie are just fine—just keep the servings small for the whole family (portion control is key in preventing excessive weight gain). You do not need to serve dessert with every dinner.

Do not decide that your child "does not like" any specific food before he is an adult.

All tastes are learned! We are born with a preference for sweet and salt tastes, so that we will *want* to drink breast milk as newborns. Other than that we learn our food likes and dislikes. Breastfed children actually learn to like the foods that their mothers eat, because flavors come through in the milk.

If children are offered specific foods on a regular basis, most will eventually enjoy them. Some people have more sensitive taste buds—they taste foods more intensively than others do. This can lead to aversions to strong-tasting and strong-smelling foods. Still, frequent exposure to foods can overcome many aversions. Children may not like spicy-hot foods—tolerance for hot spices builds over time. However, do not rule out highly flavored foods.

Remember, children eventually eat whatever their families eat, if that is what they are given. In India, children eat Indian foods; in Thailand, they eat Thai foods. American families eat a wide variety of ethnic and regional foods. Never rule a food out—your child may surprise you with what he decides he likes.

Actions for the week
choose one or two that you are not already doing

1. Think about ways you could put more structure into your children's eating habits and experiment with something new.
   - Have your child sit down at the table for all meals and snacks.
   - Offer only water between meals and snacks.
2. Think about your interactions with your child at meal and snack times and make some changes.
   - Do not react when your child does not eat as much as you think he should at a meal.
   - Do not clap and celebrate when your child eats something new.
   - Engage your child in conversation about anything other than whether or not he is eating.
3. Prepare meals for the whole family rather than being a short-order cook, catering to specific likes/dislikes.
   - Put very small amounts of each food on your child's plate.
   - Allow him to eat what he wants of what you have prepared for the meal.
   - Use the "three strikes and you're out" rule to deal with tantrums, whining, or complaining about what is served—don't let one child disrupt the meal for the whole family.

What Should Parents Be Eating?

F IFTEEN-YEAR-OLD JULIE and her mom came to see me about Julie's weight issue. We talked about what Julie typically ate for meals and snacks and what was served at family meals. Mom said that she rarely fixed vegetables by themselves, because she really didn't like them. She made salads from iceberg lettuce, without much else, because that was what she was used to, and the family ate a lot of boxed or processed foods.

We started working on ideas for healthy, delicious, and vegetable-centered recipes during Julie's weight management sessions, and we toured a grocery store to find healthy alternatives for some of the family's favorite foods.

Julie's mom just needed to find some tasty ways to enjoy vegetables, and Julie was an easy sell. Their eating habits improved, and Julie lost some of her excess weight.

● ● ● ● ● ● ● ● ● ● ● ● ●

What we as parents eat is the biggest influence on our kids' food choices. Yes, almost any kid will eat candy, chips, and fries and guzzle high-sugar drinks given the opportunity. But they can only learn to eat fruits, vegetables, whole grains, and other healthy foods if we are eating those foods and

> We are all faced with a series of great opportunities brilliantly disguised as impossible situations.
> —Charles Swindoll

offering the same fare to them. By being concerned about our own nutritional status and health, we show our children the importance of healthy choices without ever saying a word!

What is important for adults?

Eating a healthy diet and keeping physically active are the two most important lifestyle behaviors that we parents can model for our children. Adults typically gain one and eight-tenths to two pounds every year after about eighteen years of age. There are a variety of factors that cause this, but mainly we tend to move less, without decreasing our calorie intake.

In high school we may have walked or biked to and from school and activities, played on a sports team, or had an active job that required standing on our feet or moving constantly (restaurant dishwasher, grocery bagger, babysitter). When we left high school for a full-time job or college, our sports participation most likely ended, our job may have been less active, we may have had a car . . . you get the idea—we did not need to move as much.

Did we reduce our food intake in proportion to our lessened activity? In most cases, if we did not make an effort to stay physically active and/or to decrease our calorie intake, our weight began to creep up—not enough to get excited about in any one year, but oh my, by age thirty we might have begun feeling kind of thick around the middle.

Once we became parents, we may have had the added stress of exhaustion—work all day, take care of kids at night. Stay-at-home parents don't really have it any easier than those who work full-time outside the home. Being home with young children is a nonstop job—your hands are always wet from changing diapers, preparing food, cleaning up food, giving baths.

Exhaustion tends to make us hungry—we keep eating, thinking that food will give us a boost. That results in more weight gain! If you are always tired, maybe you are not getting enough sleep. We want to make sure our kids are getting sleep, which means that we need to model getting enough sleep—this also has an effect on our weight (check out chapter 9 on the importance of sleep).

And then there is the weight gain that comes with pregnancy and needs to come off after the baby is born. Everyone said you were "all baby," "hadn't gained anything anywhere else on your body"—you found that to be a big lie when you tried to put on a pre-pregnancy pair of jeans!

Whenever I take care of friends' young kids now, I realize that young parents are way too hard on themselves. It is tiring and darn hard to get anything done, even with one baby or toddler around, let alone two or more children.

Go back to chapter 2 and remind yourself to eat a balanced diet that includes whole grains, fruits and vegetables, lean protein sources, and low or nonfat dairy products or dairy substitutes. Read appendix 1 for detailed information on how much of each food group we need and what each group provides. If our children see us eating a balanced diet, they will think of that as "normal." Conversely, if our kids see us eating a lot of junk and not much in the way of fruits, veggies, whole grains . . . they will see that as what adults eat, regardless of what we try to feed them!

Review chapter 1 and think about how *you* eat—are you eating on the run, eating while you work, skipping meals, grazing all evening? If so, apply the recommendations in that chapter to yourself. By not taking the time to take care of yourself, you are telling your kids that caring for yourself is not truly important. By the time they reach their teenage years, they will be copying your behavior.

I recently worked with a delightful, high-achieving high school senior, Katherine, whose mother was concerned about her overall nutrition. Katherine was a vegetarian, and both she and her mom thought that she was not truly meeting her nutritional needs. An injury also had prevented Katherine from playing sports for the previous two years, which had resulted in some excess weight gain. Katherine's mom was a busy professional who was struggling to balance home and work. Katherine had picked up on her mom's way of skipping breakfast or just eating a quick piece of toast in the morning. She worked on school projects through lunch period and then ate whatever was available after school. She was not always home for family dinners because of her busy schedule of activities, so she snacked late in the evening while doing homework.

Always on the run, Katherine ate a lot of cheese for protein, rather than healthier vegetarian options of beans and whole grains; she often did not eat a balanced meal all day. If her eating style doesn't change, Katherine will be very overweight and quite malnourished by the time she is thirty. She will also be malnourished due to not eating a balanced diet.

Where did these habits come from? Bottom line—she learned her chaotic eating habits by watching her mother's chaotic eating habits.

Actions for the week
choose one or two that you are not already doing

1. Look at "how" you are eating and see if you need to make any changes: Do you need to start eating breakfast, sit down when you eat, quit eating while you work?

2. Review "what" you are eating: Do you need to eat more vegetables or fruits? Do you need to drink more milk or get more calcium?

3. Look at how your children eat—are they copying your less healthy eating habits? If so, start making changes.

4. What can you do to increase physical activity? Try walking fifteen minutes a day. If you are already walking, running, or doing some form of exercise, try increasing the amount of time or the number of days you work out.

5. Keep track of the number of hours that you are sedentary (at the computer, watching TV, reading, and so on). Decrease your sedentary time and increase your active time by one hour per week, to start.

• • • • • • • • • • • • • • Part Three

Universal Issues

My Child's Weight Is Out of Control —What Should I Do?

R YAN WAS A FIVE-YEAR-OLD WHO WEIGHED NINETY-SEVEN pounds when his parents brought him to see me, up from eighty-four pounds five months earlier. He was a very active preschooler, but he loved to eat! By making some changes in eating and continuing his activity, his weight gain slowed, but it was still increasing at a higher than normal rate. At six-and-a-half years old, Ryan's weight was 112 pounds and his height fifty-five inches—he was the height of a normal ten-year-old and the weight of a fourteen-year-old. He was growing faster than normal in both weight and height; the good news was that his body mass index (BMI, or ratio of weight to height) had actually decreased over the previous year and a half.

The changes in his eating were paying off—however, he was still always hungry. He was tested at a university medical center for every genetic and hormonal abnormality known to cause obesity—all the tests were normal. That was actually frustrating for his parents. Why did Ryan have this problem? Why couldn't his appetite ever be satisfied? What did this mean for his future?

● ● ● ● ● ● ● ● ● ● ● ● ● ●

Ryan was one of many children I have seen in my practice who have serious problems with excessive weight gain. We know that excess weight gain is due to eating more calories than we burn off with activity, but we do not fully understand all of the factors that affect our appetite and how our bodies process extra energy.

Jim's mother, Joanne, called me one day for help. Her son had had a voracious appetite all of his life. He was a normal-sized newborn, seven and a half pounds; by one year of age his weight had increased from the fiftieth percentile to the seventy-fifth percentile. No big deal—lots of kids change percentiles for weight or length over the first year. Jim "ate like there was no tomorrow" from the time he was six months old and started solid foods. By eighteen months his weight was up to the ninetieth percentile—this was a bit of a red flag. Most kids actually "thin out" a little after a year of age, when they begin walking, but Jim was tall, so no worries. By two years, his weight was well above the ninety-fifth percentile for age and was quickly skyrocketing out of control; soon, the mark for his weight was off the chart.

His mother told me that doctors said that he would grow out of his overweight—he was just a big kid. By eight years of age, Jim was weighing in at about 180 pounds. His doctor sent him to an endocrinologist (who deals with hormone abnormalities) to see if this weight gain was due to low thyroid or some other hormonal problem—all the tests came back normal. The family was trying to watch what they ate and keep Jim active. Jim was hungry all the time and would eat huge amounts of food, given the chance.

By eleven years of age, he weighed 287 pounds, and when he came to see me he was twelve years old and weighing over 300 pounds (his pediatrician's office scale did not go over 300 pounds, so that is what they recorded). Jim was weighing in once a week at a local gym, where he was working with a physical trainer to find ways to safely exercise—his highest weight recorded there was 315 pounds. He was very tall for his age, but his BMI was over fifty—in the super-obese range for anyone at any age.

Jim was not a sit-on-the-couch-and-eat-potato-chips-all-day kind of kid. He was bright, did well in school, and played sports at least two or three seasons of the year. His family was fairly active—his mom was overweight, but not to the point that Jim was. His dad was a little overweight, but in fairly good shape. Jim hated being different! He hated being "fat." His parents moved him to a private school in fifth grade because of the teasing and harassment he got for his size in public school. He was quite willing to learn new ways of eating and to work on being more active, but this was hard—he was still hungry all the time.

We all know people who seem to eat and eat and eat and remain thin as beanpoles. We also know individuals who eat a lot and are overweight. We see very overweight people and immediately judge them as overeaters or "lazy." Parents are judged as incompetent if they have "obese" kids, especially if they are allowing their kids to eat something "fattening"—chips, soda pop, ice cream, candy. Kids who are very overweight are often teased and picked on as they get older. I've watched teenagers joke about their own weight, but I believe it is often just a way to deflect the teasing and judgment they have had to put up with for years.

What can a parent do?

Be aware of your child's weight and "weight-for-length ratio" starting from infancy. When you are at well-baby appointments, ask your physician or nurse to turn the growth chart over and plot the weight-for-length ratio. A high ratio is not a problem if it is staying on the same percentile—if the percentile starts increasing, it is time watch more closely. After your child is two years of age, look at his BMI, and make sure it is plotted on the growth chart.

If your child's weight-for-length ratio or BMI increases beyond the eighty-fifth percentile, start getting weight and height measurements a little more often. If the ratio levels off, no worries, but what if it continues to rise, like Jim's and Ryan's did?

Do not restrict your child's eating or put your child on a diet! I cannot say this more emphatically. If we do not let our kids eat enough to feel full, we are asking for them to start sneaking food when we are not looking—and that food will not be the type we want them to eat.

Do offer foods that are lower in calorie density than traditional foods but are still filling. Following the tips in the "Flavorful Low-Calorie Substitutes" section reduces calories of traditional foods by anywhere from 18 percent to 38 percent. That may not seem like much, but by eating only a hundred calories per day more than our bodies need, a child or adult will gain an extra ten pounds in one year. Small changes definitely add up! Many parents look at me cross-eyed when I make these recommendations—"My child would never go for vegetables cooked into their rice or potatoes." Time and time again, I see kids eat these types of foods when they come to see me and we cook together.

Do have desserts occasionally, but serve them in very small dishes. You don't have any small dessert bowls? Use small teacups or go to a thrift store and see what you can find. When you use small dessert bowls, you cannot fit more than about three ounces of ice cream in them—a great "company" dessert is three ounces or one-third cup of ice cream topped with a few slices of strawberry or a few raspberries and a drizzle (one to two teaspoons) of chocolate sauce (165 calories). If this is served in a teacup or a small bowl, it looks like plenty; if it is put in a cereal bowl, it looks like almost nothing!

When you buy ice cream, consider buying a pint at a time rather than a half-gallon. Yes, it may be more expensive, but what is more harmful—eating all of that less expensive half-gallon of ice cream, or spending more money but limiting your family to reasonable serving sizes?

Try making pudding from a mix using nonfat milk (it works, even if the package says it won't). Pour the pudding into individual custard dishes that have been partially filled with berries, canned pineapple, peaches, banana, or other fruit. Chill in the refrigerator. By mixing pudding with fruit, you can stretch a package meant to serve four to serve eight—again, use those small dessert bowls or teacups to serve it in. If you make a cake or a pie or cookies, put small servings on individual plates and freeze the rest for a later date. Desserts are not a problem *if* they are doled out in small servings, and they are not sitting around to be tempting. Chapter 13 has more ideas for healthy desserts for you and your kids to try.

Set basic standards for how your family and children eat

Require that all meals and snacks are eaten while sitting at the table without television, books, or toys.

Flavorful Low-Calorie Substitutes

- One-half cup of nonfat plain yogurt sweetened with one teaspoon jam has about 75 calories, whereas one-half cup of lowfat flavored yogurt has about 120 calories.

- One cup of sliced apple has about 55 calories, whereas one cup of apple juice has 120 calories.

- One small chicken leg (two ounces of meat) baked without the skin has about 107 calories; the same size chicken leg roasted with the skin has about 130 calories.

- Cook rice with lots of vegetables. Combine one-half cup of rice with one cup of chicken, beef, or vegetable broth; about three-quarters through the cooking time (check directions on package for time), add two cups of chopped raw vegetables such as broccoli, bell peppers, onions, mushrooms, zucchini, and/or celery. Allow rice to finish cooking while the vegetables are steaming—add a little extra water or broth if the pan gets dry before the rice is done. You'll cut the calories to about 70 for each one-half cup serving versus 110 calories for one-half cup of plain cooked rice.

- Dice one large potato and steam in a covered saucepan; after about ten to fifteen minutes, add one cup of finely diced fresh or frozen broccoli, zucchini, onion, and/or any other vegetables you have on hand. When the potato and the vegetables are soft, mash them together with seasonings such as garlic or garlic powder, pepper, and paprika and one-fourth cup nonfat milk. This will make a total of about three cups—115 calories per cup versus 150 calories per cup of plain mashed potatoes (without butter).

Chapter 13 gives more ideas for reducing calories in recipes that we commonly prepare.

Eat with your kids—family meals are extremely important for improving nutrition.

Serve vegetables and/or fruit at every meal.

Make sure that your family is eating whole grains. High in fiber and more nutritious, they are also more filling than refined "white grains" (white rice, white pasta, white bread).

Drink nonfat or one-percent milk as well as water. Sugared drinks, juices, and soda pop are all very high in calories with little to no nutritional value! Dress up your water once in a while by adding sliced lemons or limes.

Seeing is believing

Find ways to make food look as if it is enough to satisfy the appetite—your overweight child will take less food without anyone saying a word. The whole family benefits from these ideas.

Apply the idea for smaller dessert dishes above to all dishes. Invest in smaller plates and bowls and glasses. Dishes and glasses have increased in size by about 36 percent since the 1960s. When we have a bigger plate, we think we need more food on it to be satisfied. What looks like a normal serving size on an eight-inch plate looks like an appetizer on a twelve-inch plate. A cup of milk looks reasonable in a ten-ounce glass but looks like very little in a sixteen-ounce tumbler. There are several research studies that show us that people eat considerably more food when they eat from bigger dishes.

Learn everything you can,
anytime you can,
from anyone you can
—there will always come a time
you will be grateful you did.
—Sarah Caldwell

Use smaller serving containers. If we see a giant bowl or pan of mashed potatoes, we will definitely take more than if we see a small bowl or saucepan full of mashed potatoes—and we will not even realize we are doing this! How much do you scoop out of a pint container of ice cream versus a two-gallon tub of ice cream? Cereal, chips, meat, and bread are all available in very large packages these days—the "value packs." We tend to give ourselves more or prepare larger amounts for our family when a food comes in a large volume.

If you buy value packs, try repackaging food into smaller containers before putting them away. If there is no difference in price, buy smaller packages of food (especially items such as meat or cheese).

What about eating out?

These ideas work very well at home, but what about when we eat out? Restaurants lure you in by offering large serving sizes—the "all-you-can-eat spaghetti, pancakes, ribs, buffet . . . bottomless fries and soda pop." It is not uncommon for a restaurant meal to top 2,000 calories; it is difficult to get a complete meal under 1,000 calories. Large serving sizes as well as increased fat, sugar, and salt in restaurant foods are all culprits in tempting us to eat more than we need.

Consider these alternatives for your family:

- Splitting meals between two family members.
- Ordering a salad and an appetizer, rather than a whole entree.
- Getting "to go" boxes at the beginning of a meal and putting half of each person's meal in a box for the next night's dinner, before you start eating.
- If going out for fast food, try a sub sandwich shop rather than a burger-and-fries place. Order the sandwiches without mayonnaise to cut out 100–150 calories; consider splitting a twelve-inch sandwich between two people.
- If you are going to a burger place, get a burger and salad and water or milk for each person and one order of fries for all to share.
- If you are going out for pizza, either order a pizza that will give each person only one or two pieces, or order pizza by the slice. Each slice of a "medium" pizza is anywhere from 200 to 450 calories, depending on the actual size of the pizza and its toppings; add extra calories for stuffed crusts, extra cheese, or several meats. Go for the thin-crust pizzas with vegetables and no more than one type of meat. Soon, most chain restaurants will be required to post the calories in their menu items, which will be very helpful in figuring out how to get the taste you want, without getting more calories than you want.

Keep moving!

Turn off the electronics. In chapter 3, "Kids Are Made to Be Active," we stressed the importance of limiting sedentary activities. If kids cannot watch television, play video games, or play games on the computer, they will find something to do that is likely to get them moving just a little.

Work on getting your child to play actively. It can be very difficult to get your overweight child to go outside and play—the more your child sits around, the more weight she will gain; the more weight she gains, the more difficult it will be for her to play actively with other kids and the more she will be self-conscious about her ability to run fast, shoot baskets, ride a bike. Excess weight gain turns into a vicious cycle; it is hard to know which came first, the difficulty in moving around or the weight gain, but they both build on each other.

When you are home, go out and walk or ride bikes or shoot baskets with your child. If you are working when he gets home from school or during the summer, consider a program like the Boys & Girls Club or other after-school and summer program so that he is not sitting at home watching television.

There are many things that parents can do to help overweight or even obese kids to slow their weight gain. All of the above ideas and the information in previous chapters will help. But there is no magic bullet—excessive weight gain is caused by both environment and genetics (more on this topic in chapter 11). We know that our environment, which promotes overeating of high-calorie food, is the biggest contributor; everywhere in the world where high-calorie foods are abundant, there is a growing problem with obesity.

This problem has increased drastically over the past thirty years. That is both good and bad news—the good news is that we can alter our environment to decrease obesity; the bad news is that we have created a toxic environment that is causing us to gain weight excessively, which is in turn making us sick—more diabetes, heart disease, stroke, cancers.

Actions for the week

choose one or two that you are not already doing

1. Buy smaller plates and bowls for serving meals.
2. Try some new recipes that lower the caloric density of your child's favorite foods.
3. Start eating all meals and snacks at the table.
4. Eat together as a family at least three times this week (gradually increase to at least once a day).
5. Try splitting meals or putting half of your and your child's meals in "to go" boxes before you start eating at a restaurant.
6. Order salads with your burgers at fast-food restaurants.
7. Spend one or two days without any TV, video, or computer games.
8. Find an activity that your child might enjoy and sign him up—arts and crafts, choir, music lessons, swimming lessons, sports—anything that gets him out of the house and on his feet.

What Does Getting Enough Sleep Have to Do with My Child's Weight?

I DON'T WANT TO GO TO BED!" "I'm not sleepy!" "Mommy, I need a drink of water." "I need to go potty." "I hear a scary noise." "You forgot to wash my face!"

• • • • • • • • • • • • •

These are words we have all heard called out from our children's bedrooms. No doubt you could add to this list. Toddlers, especially, seem to fight going to sleep with a passion.

Why don't we just let them stay up until they are willing to go to bed on their own? What is the big deal about kids having an established bedtime?

Bedtime basics

All parents need some peace and quiet in the evening in order to take care of their own needs. Kids need to go to bed early enough so that it is not a struggle to get them up and going in the morning—especially if they have to be ready for daycare or school. It is not such a big deal if they can sleep until nine or ten in the morning, but it is if they have to wake up by six or seven.

Lack of sleep affects school performance and general daytime functioning; it contributes to behavior problems and increases problems related to attention deficit and hyperactivity disorder.

Another major reason for getting enough nighttime sleep is the prevention of excess weight gain and obesity. That's right—infants, toddlers, and children who do not sleep enough at night starting in infancy tend to become overweight at a much higher rate than those who do.

The excess weight or obesity in early childhood does not go away as kids get older. Adolescents who are not sleeping enough at night also tend to become more obese than their peers who are sleeping more.

So . . . just how much sleep do kids and adults need? According to the National Sleep Foundation, sleep needs vary by individuals but in general conform to these guidelines:

Age	*Need for Sleep*
Newborn infants: 0–2 months	12–18 hours (including frequent naps)
Infants: 3–11 months	14–15 hours (including 2 naps/day)
Toddlers: 1–3 years	12–14 hours (including 1 nap/day)
Preschoolers: 4–5 years	11–13 hours (including 1 nap/day)
School-age children: 6–10 years	10–11 hours
Teens: 11–17 years	At least 8½–9¼ hours
Adults	7 to 9 hours

A good amount of research has been conducted on sleep and its relationship to obesity in children. Children who get the least amount of sleep (less than nine hours for under five years, less than eight hours for five- to ten-year-olds, and less than seven hours for older children) have been shown to have a 92 percent risk of being overweight or obese.

The relationship between a good night's sleep and weight gain holds true for adults as well. It is thought that daytime napping does not make up for nighttime sleep, because the quality of daytime sleep is not the same. Nighttime sleep, over several hours, is deeper and more restorative than daytime naps. What a nice thought—a good night's sleep as part of our weight management program.

The take-home message is—get those kids (and ourselves) in bed earlier. Much easier said than done in this hectic world! Pick up kids from daycare . . . fix dinner, and have a nice family meal . . . get kids to do their homework . . . baths . . . oh, no—it is already nine PM. In order to get to work on time, drop the youngest kid off at before-school daycare, and get the older kids to the middle or high school bus on time, everyone has to be up by six-thirty AM at the latest.

Living well and beautifully and justly are all one thing.
—Socrates

Now, assuming the eight-year-old is in bed right at nine PM, she will only get nine and a half hours' sleep. The twelve-year-old, who has to write a paper and do his math homework, will be lucky to be in bed by ten-thirty, so that means seven and a half hours' sleep, and the sixteen-year-old, who has put off his homework until after dinner, will be up until midnight, so he will get only six and a half hours' sleep. It is time to do some family problem solving in the area of getting enough sleep.

Infants, toddlers, and preschoolers

Starting bedtime rituals early is important. Very young infants (birth to two months old) often have erratic sleep schedules—they have not yet developed circadian rhythms that tell them to sleep at night and be more wakeful during the day. They need more sleep than any of us—up to eighteen hours per day.

Your baby's nighttime "bedtime" should allow her to sleep eleven to twelve hours once she starts sleeping through the night. To manage this, look at the time you need to have her up in the morning to fit your schedule. Do you need to get her to daycare by seven AM, which means she needs to be awake by five-thirty or six? If so, you want to work on moving that bedtime to six-thirty or seven PM.

When your infant wakes for feeding during the night, stick to business! Just feed—don't change him unless absolutely necessary; don't turn on the light; don't talk or play games. This is nighttime, when "normal people" are sleeping. If you have a colicky baby who cries for long periods at night, do your soothing (walking, rocking, caressing) without lights on and without talking, and remember that "this too shall pass."

Once your baby shows you that he can sleep for longer periods of time, don't jump up to feed him the moment he peeps. Allow him to fuss for a few minutes. If he does not show signs of settling back down, feed him . . . but if he does, let him go back to sleep. Put your baby to bed drowsy, but awake—he needs to learn to self-soothe himself to sleep. This will pay major dividends as he gets older.

Once your baby is sleeping through the night, work on bedtime rituals—feed, rock, read a story (yes, even to a four-month-old). Some infants are sleeping through the night very well by two to four months but then around six months start waking and crying again. This is the time to pat her on the back and assure her that you are there and everything is all right—it is *not* the time to start middle-of-the-night feedings again! Do make sure that your baby has had a hearty feeding before bed—some solids (for infants over six months of age) and a good nursing or bottle within an hour of bedtime can help prevent waking due to hunger.

Toddlers and preschoolers thrive on structure. Bedtime rituals are important—take bath, put on jammies, brush teeth, read story, say prayers, and go to bed. Avoid highly stimulating, active play and television for half an hour to an hour before bedtime. We want our kids to be relaxed and ready to snuggle down and sleep when we put them to bed.

A Bedtime Story

One parent told me that when her kids were toddlers and preschoolers, her husband often "flew them into bed"—he would hold them high in the air and they would fly all over the house and then into bed, where they'd have a story, bedtime prayer, and then say good night. Granted, it was not all smooth and easy! Her older one would be all sleepy-eyed after a story and prayers; as soon as they said good night she would pop awake again and want to "talk." She didn't get out of bed—she just wanted her mom or dad to keep her company until she went to sleep; and she would whine and cry for an hour or more, especially when they kept going in to try to calm her down.

The parents finally decided that they had to put a stop to this—they told their two-and-a-half-year-old daughter that if she whined or cried, they would shut the door (leaving the nightlight on) and would not come in. If she settled down, they would leave the door open. It took a week of big-time crying and whining, but she finally gave up and went to sleep willingly.

School-age kids

Our kids begin to be more independent once they start elementary school. They can get themselves ready for bed, or they can dawdle for ages after repeatedly being told to get pajamas on and brush their teeth—you find them in their rooms playing with a toy, looking at a book, still totally dressed. It helps to have a "carrot" to get them moving—we will read an extra chapter in a book, if you are completely ready for bed by seven-fifteen PM (it helps to always have a good chapter book going for school-age kids!).

Establishing a specific bedtime that your kids know is hard and fast is important. I always like it when a child can tell me what his bedtime is—that makes it more likely that he will actually be in bed around that time. Having a ritual that you stick to most of the time is important for school-age kids as well as for toddlers and preschoolers. When you have an evening where you are out and coming home late, it can be helpful to make a plan on the way home for getting right to bed.

When my kids were young we always had at least one evening activity every week. If things went late, we'd talk with the kids about our "plan" on the drive home—they would decide whether to brush teeth or put on pajamas first. Simply having the kids verbalize what needed to happen as soon as we got home made getting them in bed much faster . . . and that meant I could get to bed on time as well.

Aim for ten and a half or eleven hours of sleep for kids in elementary school. If they need to get up by seven AM, they need to be in bed by eight or eight-thirty PM. Earlier than that sounds impossible, but if they need to be up by six-thirty they need to be in bed by seven-thirty or eight. If we aim for ten and a half or eleven hours, our kids will likely get at least the minimum of ten hours of nighttime sleep that the experts say they need.

Middle school and high school kids

Eleven- to seventeen-year-olds still require lots of sleep, but they have a hard time believing that. Just go to any middle school or high school during first period—lots of kids are having a hard time staying awake and concentrating.

These are the ages when kids become more active in things that do not involve us parents—sports, school plays, babysitting, afterschool jobs, youth groups.

It is easy for them to become overscheduled, which makes it nearly impossible for them to participate in activities, do homework, eat a family dinner, and get to bed at a reasonable time. Parents and kids need to sit down together to plan for activities—look at a schedule of each day and see where things fit. It will be necessary to choose among activities . . . all the activities are good, but doing *all* of them is not good for any child or teenager.

Think about how much homework your child has; when he is going to eat, sleep, and have family time and downtime; make logical decisions on which activities to include. If your child really wants to be in the "zero hour" jazz band (practice starting at six-thirty AM), maybe playing soccer this season is just not realistic. If running cross-country is her passion, maybe piano lessons could be suspended for the cross-country season. How many advanced or honors classes is your teenager taking, and how much afterschool homework does that involve?

If advanced classes equal not enough sleep, then maybe taking more regular classes and just one or two advanced classes is the better approach. We do our children no favors by pushing them to take more academically intense classes if the result is sleep deprivation and thus decreased school performance, increased weight gain, decreased family time, and very little downtime. We all need balance in our lives, and getting enough sleep is an important part of that.

How do we improve the quality of our kids' sleep?

We not only want to get our children to bed at a reasonable time, we want to make sure that they are getting quality sleep. According to the National Sleep Foundation, there are several practices that help:

Consistent bedtime—Children need to go to bed at about the same time every night. Even adults tend to sleep better when they go to bed and get up at the same times each day.

Positive, relaxing environment at bedtime—This is a good time for stories for younger kids or quiet reading for older kids and teens.

Turn off television and video games one-half to one hour prior to bedtime. Stimulating entertainment just prior to bedtime may make it difficult for a child to fall asleep and stay asleep. Watching violent TV shows or movies or playing video games any time during the day or evening may cause more waking from nightmares (even for older kids).

Cool, dark, quiet bedroom—Keeping your child's bedroom relatively cool, dark (a nightlight or light from the hallway should be the only light), and quiet throughout the night will help her to sleep without waking.

Avoid caffeine—Children do not need to be drinking *any* caffeinated beverages—coffee, coffee drinks, black tea, caffeinated sodas, or energy drinks. These drinks can definitely prevent good sleep, especially if consumed late in the day or in the evening. And, of course, caffeinated soda pop adds extra calories and weight gain.

Use time management techniques to get kids in bed earlier

What are your kids doing between school and when you come home from work? Sports practices, play practice, music lessons, tutoring, daycare, hanging out—is there any way that some homework could be done during that time?

What about the time between getting home and dinner? Could baths be taken, homework done?

Is the television or computer on for entertainment? Could these activities be relegated to "only if all the essentials are done" and turned off at least half an hour before bedtime?

Is dinner late because you are doing all the work? Could your kids help with food preparation, table setting, and other chores? See chapter 13 for some super-fast meals (stir-fry chicken over rice, super-fast version; macaroni and cheese—always pretty quick to make, even though it is totally from scratch; tacos; quesadillas).

Businesses frequently conduct time management studies to figure out ways to increase efficiency. We can certainly do some time studies at home—keep a log of what you and your family do before and after work or, if you are at home, how you spend your day. Then objectively look at what you really enjoy doing, what are necessary activities (grocery shopping, laundry, food preparation), and what is taking up your time that you'd rather not be doing at all.

Are there any big time-consumers that can be cut out? Are there any "necessary activities" that can be delegated to another family member or even hired out (a housecleaner or yard worker once or twice a month can be a real sanity-saver, especially when both parents are working—this may require a review of finances, but it may be well worth giving up a few dinners out to have someone else do some home maintenance). Finding some ways to decompress your schedules can make getting your kids and yourself to bed on time—and eating healthy as well—much easier.

Actions for the week
choose one or two that you are not already doing

1. Set bedtimes for your kids if you do not already have them—talk with your kids about what is reasonable.

2. Move bedtimes fifteen minutes earlier each week until you and your kids are getting recommended levels of sleep.

3. Make a rule that there will be no TV or computer games until all necessary evening chores are done (homework, dishes, room tidying, baths . . . you decide what is necessary) and then, *only* if there is time before bedtime, some TV can be watched or computer games played—and only if your child has time left in his weekly "screen time" allotment. Be sure that the TV, computer, or video games are turned off at least half an hour before bedtime, so that your child or teen has time to wind down in order to sleep well.

4. Get yourself to bed fifteen minutes earlier each night. Work backward until you are getting a *minimum* of seven hours of sleep each night. As in everything else, you need to be a role model for your kids in healthy behavior.

A Word to the Wise
About Eating Disorders

J AMIE WAS A TWELVE-YEAR-OLD GIRL suffering from full-blown anorexia nervosa when I met her when she was a patient in the hospital psychiatric unit. She was the second child in a family of high achievers. Her sister, who was five years older, was a star athlete, excellent student, and extremely beautiful. Her parents were very fit, active people who expected the best from their children. Jamie was a good student and a good athlete who put a lot of pressure on herself to perform . . . and she did not want to become overweight.

In fifth grade she started throwing away the desserts in her school lunches; later, she started discarding her whole lunch and her weight began decreasing. She ate less and less at family meals, and her further weight loss caught her parents' attention. Jamie's low weight was to the point of being life-threatening. After outpatient counseling did not help her gain weight, she was admitted to the hospital for inpatient psychiatric treatment of anorexia nervosa. With intensive therapy, nutrition support, and family counseling over two months, Jamie's weight improved and she went home. Family counseling continued for a long time.

● ● ● ● ● ● ● ● ● ● ● ● ●

It is hard to know why a child develops an eating disorder, but we know that a focus on weight at home, in school, or in the community, and obsession with perfection, as well as very controlling parents are risk factors. Research suggests that there may be a genetic predisposition to developing an eating disorder.

The most commonly found eating disorders in today's society are:

- Anorexia nervosa: a person eats so little that he is essentially starving himself—yes, this happens in boys and men as well as in girls and women. Individuals with anorexia nervosa obsess about their weight and tend to exercise to excess—weight loss becomes life-threatening.

- Bulimia nervosa: a person binges on food and then purges by vomiting, taking laxatives, or exercising excessively in an effort to get rid of the extra calories. Weight is typically normal or even a little high for persons with this disorder.

- Anorexia with bulimia: a person combines eating very little food with purging whenever she feels she has overeaten.

- Binge-eating disorder: a person frequently eats unusually large amounts of food, consuming up to 3,000 or 4,000 calories at a time. Individuals with binge-eating disorder often become extremely obese.

Recognizing eating disorders

A woman named Mary came to my office weighing 265 pounds; she had already lost 150 pounds on her own over about four years of attending meetings of Overeaters Anonymous, a twelve-step recovery program for compulsive eaters. But she had gained a little weight back and was having a very difficult time losing weight again. Mary knew that she had binge-eating disorder. She told me that when she was "on her way up the scale" she would go to McDonald's, eat a Big Mac with large fries and a milkshake (over 2,000 calories), and then go to Burger King and do it all over again (another 2,000-plus calories). Mary understood that she had been eating to deal with sexual and other physical abuse that had happened during her childhood and early adulthood. Now, she is dealing with her demons and learning to love herself and not to hurt herself with food. She is determined to get all the way down to a normal weight for her height and body type. It is a struggle every single day!

> Success is to be measured not so much by the position that one has reached in life ... as by the obstacles which he has overcome while trying to succeed.
> —Booker T. Washington

Eating disorders are most commonly diagnosed in teens and young adults but can occur at any age. The age at which children begin to deliberately focus on body image and perceived "fatness" is drifting downward at an alarming rate. Even kindergarteners put themselves on diets!

Eating disorders are life-threatening diseases that totally consume a person—all that person thinks about is either losing weight; getting food and then getting rid of it; or just getting food. People who have eating disorders are typically very secretive and are in total denial about their problem. That makes them very difficult to treat.

So . . . we definitely want to decrease obesity in children—but in working toward that goal, we risk pushing some kids into eating disorders. We want to take care of our own bodies and we want our kids to be health conscious, but we don't want to make our weight a main focus in our lives or in the lives of our children. What can we do?

We need to start with ourselves

Ask yourself the following questions:

Am I overly concerned about my weight?

Do I talk about feeling fat or looking fat in front of my kids?

Do I go on "diets" frequently?

Do I keep my BMI exceptionally low?

Do I disparage myself for the way I look?

These behaviors are signs of a disordered body image and an inappropriate approach to eating, and in some cases may be symptoms of anorexia nervosa.

Do I tend to eat treats when no one is looking?

Do I eat leftovers while I am alone, cleaning up the kitchen, after eating a very light meal?

Do I eat ice cream or cookies after everyone else goes to bed?

Do I eat treats on the way home from the grocery store when I'm alone?

These behaviors are signs of disordered eating and in severe cases of binge-eating disorder.

Do I feel the need to punish myself when I feel that I have overeaten?

Do I feel the need to purge or actually engage in purging when I have overeaten?

These behaviors are signs of disordered eating or, if actually purging, of bulimia nervosa.

Do I skip meals with the goal of losing weight?

This is disordered eating—we know that skipping meals typically results in overeating and weight gain, not in weight loss!

If you have a problem with your own body image and relationship with food or see yourself in any of the above scenarios, you would likely benefit from some professional counseling. If you need to lose weight, you want to find a program or a registered dietitian who can help you lose weight in a healthy and sustainable way. We often don't realize how much our own issues with body image or eating are projected onto our kids. Our healthy body image and mindful eating are helpful in giving our kids healthy body images and eating habits.

Helping to prevent eating disorders

As parents and caregivers, we can do a lot to help prevent eating disorders in our children and other children with whom we are in contact.

- Prepare our girls for the body changes that come with puberty—developing breasts and hips can be alarming for a young girl who has always been thin and lithe. Early puberty is a common time for eating disorders to develop.
- Help our kids to like themselves—low self-esteem often goes along with poor body image and is a risk for eating disorders. Show your child love, attention, warmth, affection, and acceptance.

- If your child seems to be depressed and/or anxious, seek help! Depression often goes hand in hand with eating disorders.

- Teach kids how to cope with stress—it is a normal part of life.

- Be aware of perfectionism, compulsiveness, or obsessiveness—people who develop anorexia nervosa are often perfectionists or have some degree of obsessive compulsive disorder.

- Keep lines of communication open—if your child feels that he can talk to you about anything, you are more likely to know if he is developing body image issues. Make sure that you spend plenty of time listening to him!

- Allow your child physical privacy as she gets older. Your child needs some control over her own body.

- Enjoy relaxing meals together.

- Discuss the futility of "diets"—we are all bombarded with magazine covers that promise "Lose Ten Pounds in Ten Days," or "Get a Flat Stomach by Bikini Season," or "Lose Belly Fat." Talk about why those headlines are false and misleading.

- Discuss the fact that our media makes artificially thin bodies seem like the norm. Talk about how the photographs of many TV stars and magazine models are digitally altered to make them look like our false ideal, or how models do horribly unhealthy things to make their stomachs look flat and waists look small (for instance, abuse laxatives, wear compressing undergarments, or starve themselves).

Out of the Mouths of Babes

Eight-year-old Calley came to see me with her mom. Calley thought she was "fat." Her mom noticed that she was a little heavier than some other kids her age, but it was Calley who wanted to see the nutritionist. When I asked her why she wanted to lose weight, this eight-year-old said, "I want to be able to look good in a bikini when we go to Mexico for spring break." Her mother had no idea that this was a driving factor in Calley's young life.

Calley had "friends" at school who had told her that she was fat; her mother was aware of the risks for eating disorders and wanted to get onto a healthy eating track for the whole family. Actually, Calley's BMI was just at the higher end of normal; indeed, she was not overweight. This is just the type of kid whom I worry about with our society's obsession with thinness.

Actions for the week

choose one or two that you are not already doing

1. Tell your children how much you love them (you can do this every day, regardless of other actions!).

2. Tell your children how much you appreciate their hard work on some job or project (appreciation doesn't depend on how the job or project turned out; praise them for the effort they made—if they made a sincere effort).

3. Spend time talking with your kids. Cooking dinner, cleaning the garage, doing the dishes or some other job with your child, or even taking one child out for a meal at a restaurant are great times to talk—just sitting down "to talk" rarely works.

4. Eat family meals and talk about each person's day.

5. Seek help for yourself if you find that you have issues with your own body image, dieting habits, or eating behavior.

6. Seek help for your child if he seems to be having problems with self-esteem, depression, and/or body image.

How Environment and Genetics
Have Created an Obese Society

S USIE IS STICK-THIN and Maggie is stocky and muscular. Both are ten years old and growing very well—neither girl is under *or* over-weight. Susie hates it when people tell her she is skinny and Maggie is distraught when kids at school say she is chubby! When you look at the girls' growth charts, Susie's weight compared to her height is at the lower end of the normal BMI range, whereas Maggie's is at the higher end. Neither girl needs to make changes to increase or decrease her weight. Now look at Susie's parents—both tall and thin. Maggie's parents are shorter and stockier. Maggie's parents both have to work at avoiding excess weight gain, while Susie's never give weight a second thought. Maggie has grandparents, aunts, and uncles who are overweight.

● ● ● ● ● ● ● ● ● ● ● ● ● ●

These girls are both growing according to their genetic potential. It might well be that if Maggie were allowed to sit in front of the TV and snack on high-calorie foods all day she would gain too much weight; under the same conditions Susie's weight might not become an issue. The ability to gain weight when we overeat and to have the appetite to eat more than we need is genetically determined to a large degree. In this case, the reason Maggie is not overweight is because she is active and does not have the opportunity to mindlessly munch on high-calorie foods—her healthy environment keeps her from becoming obese despite her genes.

Genetics and Environment

The connection between genetics and environment has been studied in the Pima Indians of Arizona for decades by the National Institute of Diabetes and Digestive and Kidney Diseases, part of the National Institutes of Health. The Pima migrated from the Sierra Madre Mountains in Mexico 2,000 years ago. Half of the Arizona population of adult Pima Indians born since World War II have type 2 diabetes, and 95 percent of those with diabetes are obese. However, in a small study of a group of Pima who still live as their ancestors did in Mexico, the incidence of type 2 diabetes was less than one in ten, and there was a very low level of obesity. After World War II, the Arizona Pima diet changed from a traditional one high in fiber and low in fat to one high in sugar, refined starches, and fat. Their lifestyle modernized as well—they began to do less physically demanding work and to have more leisure and sedentary time. Their rates of obesity and diabetes began to skyrocket with this combination of higher calorie intake and lower levels of calorie burning. The Pima proved to have a genetic predisposition for storing fat, so that they would survive during times of famine—which backfired when living in our "obesogenic" environment. The information we have from the Pima Indians in Arizona and in Mexico shows us that genetics alone do not cause obesity. We have to have both the genetics and the environment (high calories, low physical activity) for rates of obesity to increase.

Some of us have metabolisms that speed up and burn more calories when we eat more than we need—others just store any extra calories as fat. Research studies have shown that many people who are overweight or obese have higher levels of the hormones that tell us we are hungry, and they do not respond well to those hormones that tell us when we are full. If there is a tempting food available, they will eat it, even if they just finished a meal. Other people can see a really tasty treat and leave it if they have just finished a meal. In an earlier age, we would have been glad to be able to overeat and to store fat when food was plentiful—that is what would get us through a famine, or through the winter when food was scarce.

Over the past seventy-five years, at least in Western countries such as the United States, food has become more and more plentiful and less expensive. Whereas sugar and refined flour were once a luxury, they are now cheap and easily available. High-fiber whole grains and unprocessed fruits and vegetables were once the least expensive foods—they are now more expensive than many highly processed foods.

Salt was once something we valued for food preservation (think about pioneers migrating across the plains), but now we need to find ways to decrease it. Genes that increased our ability to gain weight and store fat were lifesaving in times of famine. They are now the bane of our existence and seem to be the cause of many of our ills.

Genetics and environment—
why obesity has increased in recent years

If one parent is overweight, the chance that his or her child will be overweight is increased by three times over that of a child whose parents are both normal weight. However, if both parents are obese, the chance that their child will be obese is ten times that of children whose parents are both normal weight.

Having overweight or obese parents is not an absolute sentence to obesity for a child. We can change the environment of overeating and low physical activity for our children and greatly reduce their risk of becoming overweight or obese.

We must realize what is actually causing us to be obese. Many factors in our modern society together make overeating and low physical activity common—this results in excess weight gain, especially for those of us who have a genetic predisposition to obesity. These factors have accelerated since 1980 when obesity rates in both children and adults began to soar.

Environmental factors toxic to people with a genetic predisposition to obesity

Increased serving size, which translates into excess calories

The chart lists a few restaurant foods and commercially prepared foods that have increased in typical serving size over just the past twenty years.

Food or beverage	Twenty years ago	Now
Soda pop	6½ oz. = 85 calories	20 oz. = 250 calories
French fries	2.4 oz. = 210 calories	6.9 oz. = 610 calories
Muffin	1.5 oz. = 210 calories	4 oz. = 500 calories
Bagel	3-inch = 140 calories	6-inch = 350 calories
Average cheeseburger	333 calories	590 calories
Spaghetti and meatballs	1 cup spaghetti and 3 small meatballs = 500 calories	2 cups spaghetti and 3 large meatballs = 1025 calories
Pepperoni pizza	2 slices = 500 calories	2 slices = 850 calories
Chocolate chip cookie	1½-inch diameter = 55 calories	3½-inch diameter = 275 calories
Cheesecake	3 oz. = 250 calories	6½ oz. = 640 calories

Source: http://myfooddiary.com/resources/Games/PortionDistortion_1.asp

Most of us, especially those who have higher levels of hormones that signal hunger, are going to clean our plates at a restaurant. Remember—extra food is wasted on a person's middle just as much as it is wasted when it goes into the garbage can.

Increased serving container size

We can now buy jumbo sizes of everything. It is the "economical" thing to do—supposedly. If I can get a forty-ounce box of cereal for ten cents an ounce less than the twenty-ounce box, why in the world would I buy the twenty-ounce box? Think again—whether we believe it or not, we tend to serve ourselves larger portions from the jumbo container than from the smaller one. Are we saving money, or are we just eating more than we need? Think about ice cream. According to nutritional information on the container, one serving is one-half cup (not a whole lot). If I buy a pint of ice cream, it is going to be much easier to just give each person one-half cup than if I buy a half-gallon container, let alone a big-box store's two- or three-gallon container. Add in the increase in hunger hormones and decreased sensitivity to fullness hormones in those of us with the genetic potential to become obese, and servings become even bigger!

Increased plate, glass, and bowl size

The sizes of plates, glasses, and bowls have increased by about 36 percent over the past fifty years. Let's look at ice cream again—if you are serving yourself ice cream in a large, three-cup cereal bowl, the bowl looks almost empty! Put that same half-cup serving in a small teacup and the cup is full. Three ounces of meat and one-half cup of rice or potato and one-half cup of cooked vegetables look lost on a twelve- to fourteen-inch-diameter plate, but the quantity looks like a very complete meal on an eight-inch plate. What is the person who is genetically programmed to overeat going to do when filling that big plate or bowl? She is going to fill it full!

These are just a few ways that our environment has contributed to the overeating that has helped fuel this obesity epidemic. Other things that play into this are easy access to processed foods high in sugar, salt, and fat—these foods are easy to eat and very tasty, so we tend to eat a lot of them before we feel full. If you or your child has the genes that help your body to eat more and store extra calories as fat, it is going to be *extremely difficult* to avoid becoming overweight in our society unless you consciously change your eating environment!

A hero is an ordinary individual
who finds the strength to persevere and endure
in spite of overwhelming obstacles.
—Christopher Reeve

Technology

Technology is wonderful; it has brought us computers and the Internet, giving us the ability to gather information from all over the world without ever leaving our homes. It has brought us amazing amounts of entertainment through television, videos, computer games—we and our kids can be entertained right at home, so no more "I'm bored!" Technology has brought us automobiles so that we can easily get from place to place, without spending our time walking or cycling. It has brought us washing machines and clothes dryers, dishwashers, no-wax floors, self-propelled vacuum cleaners, power lawnmowers and even riding mowers . . . so we can do our laundry and maintain our homes and yards with a minimum of time and effort.

Along with the truly wonderful advances in technology have come some downsides—because we can do so much, with so little effort, we are less active than ever before in human history. Combine this lowered expenditure of calories with our increased caloric intake and we set the stage for anyone and everyone who has the ability to store fat to become obese! And guess what—two out of three adults in the United States are overweight, and one out of three are obese. Our kids are following right behind us, with one out of three overweight and one out of six obese. The only way to turn this epidemic around is to very purposefully change our environments to decrease our caloric intake and increase our physical activity (which requires decreasing sedentary behavior).

It is important to understand that genetics plays a big role in whether or not we become overweight or obese. But our genetics are not an ironclad sentence to a lifetime of obesity. We can counteract those genes.

Actions for the week

choose one or two that you are not already doing

1. Quit blaming yourself or your lack of willpower or discipline—look at ways your environment might cause you or your child to overeat or be inactive, and then make some changes.

2. Try buying foods in smaller containers. If you buy jumbo size containers, repackage foods in small containers as soon as you get home from the grocery store. For instance, measure out enough cereal for two or three days and put it in plastic containers or bags; put one container in the cereal cupboard at a time and store the rest out of sight.

3. Put a serving-size measuring cup in containers of ready-to-eat dry foods (for example, an eight-ounce measuring cup in the container of cereal and a one-ounce measuring cup in the container of nuts).

4. Buy smaller plates, bowls, and glasses. If you already have lunch-size plates, use them in place of large dinner plates.

5. Turn off the TV and computer games—give your child a limit that does not exceed seven hours per week (less is even better).

6. Try walking or riding bikes *with your kids* to do errands that are less than a mile or two away from home.

7. Brainstorm *with your kids* on ways that your family could increase activity and decrease serving sizes of food—make it a game.

What About Calories?

I DON'T REALLY ENJOY MAKING A BUDGET or balancing my checkbook ... but if I don't, I will likely end up in trouble by the end of the month. I need to know how much money I have, in order to prioritize my spending—I definitely need to cover the basics before I spend on luxuries. Understanding the calories in foods is much like dealing with money. You need to have an idea of how many calories you need and prioritize your eating— make sure that you are eating the foods that meet your basic nutritional needs before you spend calories on candy, chips, and other "empty-calorie foods" that are devoid of real nutrition.

● ● ● ● ● ● ● ● ● ● ● ● ● ● ● ●

We can look at our bodies as a bank—we deposit energy when we eat, which we measure in calories, just as we deposit money, which we measure in dollars, into the bank. If we deposit more calories than we need, they go into an energy savings account—our fat stores. We need to maintain a certain level of fat stores to be healthy, but if we constantly eat more than we need, our fat stores become too big and we become overweight or, if our fat stores are way too big, obese.

We take calories out of our bank for basic maintenance—we breathe, our heart beats, we blink, our muscles contract and relax, and we have a number of metabolic processes going on all the time. Children withdraw additional calories for growth and

> Opportunity is missed by most people because it is dressed in overalls and looks like work.
> —Thomas Alva Edison

development. On top of our basic usage, we use calories for all the activities that we choose to do. Every movement our bodies make uses calories—the more we move, the more calories we use.

If we are eating just what we need—putting the right amount of calories into our body's bank account—we maintain our weight, and our kids gain weight and grow at a healthy rate. Likewise, if we do not eat enough—do not put enough energy into our body's bank account—we lose weight. If our kids are not eating enough, their weight gain slows, or they lose weight; if their energy intake does not pick up, their growth in height slows, and eventually the growth of their vital organs, including their brains, slows.

The above analogy is a very simple description of what calories are and how we use them. Remember, *calorie* is just the term we use to measure energy, as *dollar* is the term we use to measure money. Our bodies have a variety of ways to tell us when we need to eat more or less—different hormones make us hungry and others tell us that we are full. This system works extremely well, unless we override it, which unfortunately we do all too often in this society of fast and convenient, highly processed food.

A fine balance of foods to meet all of our nutritional needs

Foods are made up of carbohydrates, protein, and fat—each of these groups are important for our survival, and they each provide calories. We also need a variety of vitamins and minerals. We can easily meet our calorie needs without coming close to meeting all of our nutritional needs. The example below shows two meals that are very similar in caloric value—they each meet about 27 percent of a ten-year-old boy's caloric needs, but they are vastly different in their vitamin and mineral content.

Two meals of similar caloric values but vastly different nutritional values

Meal One:

   Hot dog (two-ounce wiener, enriched white bun, one tablespoon ketchup)

   Potato chips (one ounce, about twelve chips)

   Cola (eight fluid ounces)

   582 calories

Meal Two:

   Baked chicken thigh (two-ounce)

   Steamed broccoli (three spears)

   Baked sweet potato (one cup with two teaspoons butter)

   Chocolate ice cream (one-half cup)

   Two-percent milk (eight fluid ounces)

   590 calories

Percentage of nutrients needed by the average ten-year-old boy

Nutrient	Meal One: Hot Dog	Meal Two: Chicken
Calories	27%	27%
Carbohydrates	23%	20%
Protein*	43%	100%
Fat	40%	37%
Vitamin C	11%	110%
Vitamin A	1%	145%
Calcium	6%	38%
Sodium	52%	36%
Fiber	14%	43%

*Actual needs are very low; it is not uncommon for children to eat 300–400% of protein needs per day.

   This is an extreme example of the different nutritional values of different meals. Meal One contains more foods that are low in nutrients relative to calories and higher in fat and sodium, two conditions that we want to keep relatively low—this meal should definitely just be a "once in a while" meal. Meal Two contains several foods that are very high in nutrients relative to their caloric value but also includes a dessert that is high in fat and sugar—this meal, dessert and all, could make a regular appearance on our child's menu. If your child had Meal One for lunch, Meal Two, with its very high nutritional value, would be a great idea for dinner!

When we obtain our calories from a variety of foods from the basic food groups and keep intake of low-nutrient but high-calorie foods to a minimum, we typically meet all of our nutritional needs. Our hunger and fullness signals tend to work well and we maintain a healthy weight. (See chapter 2 for ideas on how to meet our nutritional needs with ordinary foods, and see appendices 1 and 2 for more specific nutrient information.)

What do we do with this information?

Now, you know what calories are—they are just our term to measure energy expenditure. Our kids need energy to grow and develop, and they need it from carbohydrates, protein, and fat. They also need lots of other nutrients. When we eat foods in their most natural states rather than processed versions of foods (that is, whole fruits versus fruit juice, brown rice versus white rice, unprocessed meats versus hot dogs or sausage), we get their calories and all of their natural nutrients with far less sugar, salt, and fat.

Whole, basic foods definitely take more time to prepare, and they take more time to eat—we eat faster and eat more calories when food is processed to the degree that it is very easy to chew and swallow. Try eating half of a medium to large apple; later (when you are hungry again) eat one-half cup of unsweetened applesauce (both about 50 calories). Which took longer to eat? Which was more satisfying?

Our food system has worked at making foods not only easy to prepare but easy to eat. On top of that, foods have been made with lots of added sugar, salt, and fat to make them extremely tasty—David Kessler calls this "super-palatable" in his book *The End of Overeating*. When foods are super-palatable and easy to eat, we can eat them very quickly, so we often eat more calories than we need in a very short time. Now, add to that our super-sized portions at restaurants and in packaged foods—that is a recipe for a pig-out!

As parents, we do not need to be calculating the calories and protein in everything that we feed our kids, but we do need to have an understanding of the caloric value of foods. I've had many people tell me that they do not think that fruit juice has many calories at all—wrong! One-hundred-percent fruit juices actually have more calories than soda pop (110 to 140 calories per cup versus 100 calories per cup—but this is not saying that soda pop is healthy!), and juices contain nowhere near as many vitamins and minerals as fresh fruit.

Many of my clients are amazed when they find out that all-natural tortilla chips, made with canola oil and no trans fat, have about 14 calories per chip—140 calories per ounce—the same as those made with unhealthy fat. Even more astounding, fat-free whole grain pita chips have about 11 calories per chip—110 calories per ounce (they may be fat-free, but they are not a low-calorie food)—whereas a whole dinner plate of carrots, bell peppers, celery, and cucumber has only about 50 calories.

There is nothing "wrong" with either type of chip; we just need to know that they are both high in calories. We would be far better off and feel much more satisfied if we had one ounce of either type of chips and a plate of raw vegetables for our snack rather than two ounces of chips.

Actions for the week
choose one or two that you are not already doing

1. Read food labels to see if the amount of calories in a food is worth the amount of protein, fiber, vitamins, and minerals in it.

2. Pair higher-calorie foods with low-calorie foods, in order to keep calories down (a snack of chips with some vegetables; a scoop of ice cream with some unsweetened berries or peaches).

3. Pair small servings of meat, poultry, or fish with whole grains, beans, and vegetables to achieve a balanced meal.

4. Try to serve "whole," unprocessed foods most of the time at home.

5. Be aware of the excessive serving sizes we get at restaurants, and consider splitting a restaurant meal between you and one (or two) of your children. The "extra plate" charge is worth it to eat less high-calorie food.

Putting It into Practice

Recipes, Meals, and Snacks

THE RECIPES IN THIS CHAPTER ARE DIVIDED INTO SERVING sizes adequate for an older child or adult. Toddlers and preschoolers may eat as little as one-eighth to one-half a serving size. It is always best to start with a little and give a child more if she asks for it. Large amounts of foods, especially new foods, are overwhelming to a small child. Starting with very small servings also results in less waste. I am not a fan of the "clean-your-plate" club, but I would rather throw away a teaspoon of food that my child refuses than a whole cup of it.

Breakfast: Quick and easy

● ● ● ● ● ● ● ● ● ● ● ● ● ● ●

Yogurt and Oats

SERVINGS: 1

⅓ cup Old-fashioned rolled oats, dry

1 cup Plain nonfat yogurt

1 cup Diced fruit or berries

Optional:
½ to ⅔ oz. Unsalted almonds or walnuts

Optional:
1 Tbsp. Ground flaxseed

Mix all ingredients together and eat.

●

VARIATION: Use ½ cup leftover cooked rice, quinoa, or other grain in place of oats.

●

NUTRITIONAL ANALYSIS: (using 1 cup frozen blueberries, and approximately 13 whole almonds): Calories: 410; Protein: 19 gm; Carbohydrates: 60 gm; Fat: 11.4 gm; Saturated fat: 1 gm; Sodium 152 mg; Dietary fiber: 8.7 gm.

Super Breakfast Shake

SERVINGS: 1

Use the ingredients for **Yogurt and Oats** above, but substitute frozen fruit for fresh fruit. Blend in a blender and you have a thick, creamy, highly nutritious breakfast shake. If you want to thin it out, add a little milk.

Fancy Oatmeal

SERVINGS: 1   Serving size: 1 cup

⅓ cup Old-fashioned rolled oats, dry

⅔ cup Water

1 pinch Salt (optional)

½ large Apple, diced

⅛ cup Walnuts, chopped (grind walnuts for children under three)

⅛ cup, packed Seedless raisins

¼ cup 1% milk, warmed

1 Tbsp. Brown sugar

Bring water to a boil in a medium-sized saucepan. Add oats, salt, apple, walnuts, and raisins. Cook for 5–8 minutes, then cover and let sit for 3–4 minutes and serve. Top with ¼ cup warm milk and 1 Tbsp. brown sugar.

●

VARIATION: Use any hot cereal (e.g., Multigrain, Roman Meal, Zoom) or cooked grain (e.g., brown rice, quinoa, wheat bulgur, spelt) in place of oats.

●

NUTRITIONAL ANALYSIS FOR WHOLE RECIPE: Calories: 375; Protein: 8.5 gm; Carbohydrates: 55 gm; Fat: 13 gm; Saturate fat: 1.7 gm; Cholesterol: 3 mg; Sodium: 180 mg; Dietary fiber: 7 gm.

Veggie and Egg Scramble or Omelet

SERVINGS: 1 OR 2

EGG SCRAMBLE: Heat heavy frying pan. Add olive oil and vegetables. Sauté until vegetables are soft. Mix eggs with milk in small bowl and beat with a fork until mixed well; add optional seasonings as desired. Pour egg mixture into pan with vegetables and scramble until eggs are solid.

OMELET: Use water in place of milk when mixing eggs. Heat heavy frying pan, add olive oil, add eggs; as eggs start becoming solid, add vegetables and cover pan so that vegetables will steam. When eggs are set, use spatula to fold omelet in half. If vegetables are not appearing soft, add a little water to the side of the pan, cover again to allow vegetables to continue to steam for 1–2 minutes. Remove lid, allow water to evaporate, and slide omelet out of pan onto plate.

2 large Eggs
2 Tbsp. 1% milk
1 Tbsp. Olive oil
⅛ medium Onion, finely chopped
¼ medium Green or red bell pepper, finely chopped
4 medium Mushrooms, sliced
¼ cup Broccoli, finely chopped
and/or
1 cup Spinach, raw

Optional seasonings: chili powder, Tabasco sauce, cumin, cayenne pepper, salt, and black pepper to taste

Optional:
2–4 Tbsp. Grated cheese

NUTRITIONAL ANALYSIS FOR WHOLE RECIPE WITH CHEESE: Calories: 395; Protein: 21; Carbohydrates: 10 gm; Fat: 32 gm; Saturated fat: 10; Cholesterol: 460 mg; Sodium: 402 mg; Dietary fiber: 1 gm.

NUTRITIONAL ANALYSIS FOR WHOLE RECIPE WITHOUT CHEESE: Calories: 285; Protein: 14 gm; Carbohydrates: 7 gm; Fat: 23 gm; Saturated fat: 5 gm; Cholesterol: 430 mg; Sodium: 212 mg; Dietary fiber: 1 gm.

REDUCED CALORIE AND FAT VERSION OF VEGGIE AND EGG SCRAMBLE OR OMELET: If you want to decrease the calories and fat, but keep the same volume, mix 1 egg with 3 egg whites; spray pan with cooking spray, rather than using olive oil; and use just 2 tablespoons grated cheese; include all the veggies.

NUTRITIONAL ANALYSIS: Calories: 202; Protein: 22 gm; Fat: 9 gm; Saturated fat: 4 gm; Cholesterol: 230 mg.

TOAST with 1 tsp. butter and 2 tsp. jam (breads vary widely, depending on weight of slice; this assumes a 38-gm slice of 100% whole-grain bread, toasted).

NUTRITIONAL ANALYSIS: Calories: 140; Protein: 4 gm; Carbohydrates: 25 gm; Fat: 5 gm; Saturated fat: 2.7 gm: Cholesterol: 30 mg; Sodium: 209 mg; Dietary fiber: 3 gm.

NUTRITIONAL ANALYSIS FOR WHOLE BREAKFAST (egg scramble/omelet plus toast): 342 to 535 calories and 18 to 25 gm protein (depending on whether you use the regular or low-calorie version and add cheese).

Whole-Grain Toast with Peanut Butter and Jam or Honey

SERVINGS: 1

1 **38-gm slice 100% whole-grain bread, toasted**

1 **Tbsp. Natural peanut butter (you have to stir it to mix in the oil)**

2 **tsp. Jam**

or

1 **tsp. Honey**

NUTRITIONAL ANALYSIS: Calories: 200; Protein: 8 gm; Carbohydrates: 28 gm; Fat: 9 gm; Saturated fat: 1 gm; Sodium: 210 mg; Dietary fiber: 4 gm. Eat with a piece of fruit and a glass of milk for a complete, very quick meal!

Bran Flakes with Muesli, Blueberries, Almonds, Milk, and Yogurt

SERVINGS: 1

¾ **cup Bran flakes**

¼ **cup Muesli**

½ **cup Nonfat plain yogurt**

½ **cup Nonfat or 1% milk**

1 **cup Blueberries, frozen**

2 **Tbsp. Sliced almonds**

(grind for children under three)

NUTRITIONAL ANALYSIS: Calories: 420; Protein: 18 gm; Fat: 8 gm, Saturated fat: 0.5 gm, Carbohydrates: 75 gm; Sodium: 420 mg; Dietary fiber: 12 gm.

Shredded Wheat with Puffed Kamut, Banana, Nuts, and Milk

SERVINGS: 1

NUTRITIONAL ANALYSIS: Calories: 530; Protein: 21 gm; Fat: 20 gm; Saturated fat: 2 gm; Carbohydrates: 82 gm; Sodium: 140 gm; Dietary fiber: 10 gm.k

1 cup Spoon-size shredded wheat biscuits

1 cup Puffed kamut or puffed wheat

½ large Banana, sliced

¼ oup Walnuts, ohopped (grind for children under three)

1 cup Nonfat or 1% milk

Cheerios, Plain with Some Flavored Cheerios to Sweeten

SERVINGS: 1

This cereal does not supply enough calories to keep a child going all morning at school (we want kids to eat 20 to 30% of their needs at breakfast—for the average active ten-year-old, who needs about 2,150 calories per day, breakfast should provide 430 to 650 calories). Bump it up by adding a slice of toast with peanut butter (see **Whole-Grain Toast with Peanut Butter and Jam or Honey** above) or add ¼ cup chopped almonds, walnuts, or peanuts, or a couple of slices of cheese.

1½ cup Plain Cheerios

¼ cup Honey Nut Cheerios

1 medium, or

¾ cup Peach, fresh or frozen, sliced

½ cup Nonfat or 1% milk

NUTRITIONAL ANALYSIS: Calories: 275; Protein: 11 gm; Fat: 2 gm; Carbohydrates: 44 gm; Cholesterol: 3 mg; Sodium: 400 mg; Dietary fiber: 5 gm.

Lunch: Simple and nutritious

Add a fruit, raw vegetables, a small cookie or treat, and milk or water to any of the cold or hot items below to make a complete, wholesome lunch.

Be sure to pack lunch in an insulated container with an ice pack or frozen water bottle to keep things cold and safe until lunchtime!

LEFTOVER BAKED CHICKEN

1 or 2 baked, chilled chicken legs (amount depends on size and appetite of child) and whole-grain crackers.

CHEESE, MEAT, AND CRACKERS

String cheese; leftover chicken, pork, or beef slices; and whole-grain crackers.

SANDWICHES AND WRAPS

Use whole-grain bread or tortillas (whole-grain tortillas are nice because they travel well).

Traditional—still as good as ever: peanut butter and jam. Peanut butter or almond butter and thinly sliced banana.

Turkey or other meat, a slice of cheese, and thinly sliced cucumber and tomato with mayonnaise and mustard.

Egg Salad

SERVINGS: 1 OR 2

2 large Eggs, hardboiled
2 tsp. Prepared mustard
1 Tbsp. Low-fat mayonnaise
1 Tbsp. Yogurt, plain, nonfat
¼ cup Alfalfa sprouts
¼ cup Carrot, grated

NUTRITIONAL ANALYSIS FOR WHOLE RECIPE:
Calories: 230; Protein: 14 gm; Carbohydrates: 8 gm; Fat: 15 gm; Saturated fat: 4 gm; Cholesterol: 429 mg; Sodium: 428 mg; Dietary fiber: 1 gm.

ALTERNATIVE TO MAYONNAISE AND YOGURT:
Creamy Salad Dressing or Dip, in salad dressing and dip section.

Traditional Tuna Salad

SERVINGS: 2

Mix tuna, egg, mayonnaise, yogurt, relish, and celery together; place ½ mixture with lettuce on bread or in tortilla or on top of a bed of lettuce.

VARIATIONS: Use other canned or leftover fish, chicken, or turkey in place of tuna. Add in grated carrots, chopped bell peppers, chopped onion, and grated apples or chopped grapes in place of pickle relish.

1 **5-oz. can Tuna, in water, drained**
1 **large Egg, hardboiled, chopped**
1 **Tbsp. Low-fat mayonnaise**
1 **Tbsp. Yogurt, plain, nonfat**
1 **Tbsp. Sweet pickle relish**
¼ **cup Celery, finely chopped**
½ **cup Romaine lettuce, chopped**

NUTRITIONAL ANALYSIS FOR ½ RECIPE (WITH-OUT BREAD): Calories: 174; Protein: 25 gm; Carbohydrates: 5 gm; Fat: 6 gm; Saturated fat: 1 gm; Cholesterol: 134 mg; Sodium: 440 mg.

Leftover Meat with Neufchatel Cheese

SERVINGS: 1

Neufchatel cheese is a natural cheese that is very similar to cream cheese but has 33% less fat and 25% fewer calories.

Wrap a thin slice of meat around a tablespoon of cheese and then wrap that in romaine or green leaf lettuce; eat with crackers. Or spread cheese on tortilla, place meat on cheese, add vegetables, and roll up for a wrap. Or spread cheese on bread, add meat and lettuce, tomato, sliced cucumber, and sprouts for a sandwich.

2 **Tbsp. Neufchatel cheese**
2 **oz. Leftover beef, turkey, chicken, or pork, thinly sliced**
Lettuce, spinach, tomato, cucumbers, sprouts as desired

NUTRITIONAL ANALYSIS FOR MEAT AND CHEESE: Calories: 174; Protein: 18 gm; Fat: 10 gm; Saturated fat: 6 gm; Cholesterol: 65 mg; Sodium: 143 mg.

Beans, Avocado, Tomato, and Cheese

SERVINGS: 1

½ cup Black, pinto, red, or
   kidney beans, whole or
   nonfat refried beans
¼ medium Avocado, sliced
¼ medium Tomato, diced
2 Tbsp. Shredded sharp
   cheddar cheese,
   as desired

Optional:
Lettuce, chopped or torn
as desired
Salsa, tomato or mango

WRAP: Mash beans with fork or potato masher or use refried beans and spread on tortilla, add other ingredients, and roll up (heat or eat cold). **SALAD:** Whole beans are best; sprinkle beans over bed of lettuce, add avocado, tomato, cheese, and salsa as desired, and enjoy.

NUTRITIONAL ANALYSIS (without optional ingredients or tortilla): Calories: 255; Protein: 12 gm; Carbohydrates: 26 gm; Fat: 12 gm; Saturated fat: 4 gm; Cholesterol: 15 mg; Sodium: 102 mg (if beans are cooked from dry, no added salt); 562 mg (if canned beans, varies depending on brand); Dietary fiber: 12 gm. Add 100 to 150 calories for one whole-wheat tortilla.

Dinner: Healthy and convenient

Baked Greek Chicken

SERVINGS: 2   Serving size: 2 breast quarters

Remove skin from chicken and cut chicken breasts into quarters (smaller pieces will absorb more flavor from the wine, garlic, and herbs); place in baking pan. Mix olive oil, garlic, onion, wine, pepper, lemon juice, parsley, and basil together and pour over chicken. Sprinkle crumbled feta cheese over chicken. Cover pan with foil. Preheat oven and bake covered at 375 degrees for 30–40 minutes; remove foil and bake for another 20–30 minutes, or until chicken is well done.

SERVING SUGGESTION: Serve over brown rice or baked potato with steamed vegetables on the side. Or serve with sliced fruit and crackers for a quick, low-cost meal.

3 **whole Chicken breasts** (bone-in or boneless)
2 **Tbsp. Olive oil**
3 **cloves or 3 tsp. Garlic, chopped or crushed**
½ **medium Onion, chopped**
1 **cup Dry white wine** (e.g., Chablis) **or low-sodium chicken broth**
⅛ **tsp. Ground black pepper**
2 **Tbsp. Lemon juice**
¼ **cup Fresh parsley, chopped**

Optional:
Fresh basil, chopped
¼ **lb. Reduced-fat feta cheese, crumbled**

SUPER EASY VARIATIONS:

Set oven at 375 degrees. Spray baking pan with cooking spray.

- **VARIATION ONE:** Place 2 cups of dry, quick-cooking brown rice in the bottom of baking pan. Use boneless, skinless thinly sliced chicken breasts and/or thighs; arrange on top of the rice. Sprinkle with Italian seasoning, onion powder, garlic powder, olive oil, and crumbled feta cheese. Pour 2 cups water or chicken broth and 1 cup white wine or water over the whole dish and bake, covered tightly with foil, for 30 minutes. Remove cover; add 1 bag of frozen vegetables (e.g., broccoli, carrots, and cauliflower) to pan, cover again, and cook for an additional 15 minutes—this gives you a complete meal in one pan!
- **VARIATION TWO:** Slice 3 large potatoes, sweet potatoes, or yams in thin pieces. Place on the bottom of the pan. Add chicken and spices, crumbled feta cheese, and oil as in main recipe above; pour 1 cup wine or broth over

the whole dish. Bake covered for 45 minutes; remove cover and bake for an additional 15 minutes.

• **VARIATION THREE:** Put all ingredients in Variation Two in crockpot or slow cooker in the morning and cook (8 to 10 hours on low or 4 to 5 hours on high).

• **SOUP FROM LEFTOVERS:** Remove chicken from bones; put chicken, leftover juices, and vegetables in large saucepan. Add fresh celery, onion, peppers, carrots, or other vegetables (you can also just add frozen mixed vegetables), and fresh or dried parsley or basil. Add low-sodium chicken broth to get desired volume. Bring to a boil and simmer for 30–40 minutes, until fresh vegetables are soft. Add whole-grain noodles (any kind) or leftover rice and continue to cook until noodles are done.

NUTRITIONAL ANALYSIS FOR 1/6 OF RECIPE, INCLUDING BROTH: Calories: 260; Protein: 31 gm; Carbohydrates: 2.6 gm; Fat: 10.3 gm; Saturated fat: 3.2 gm; Sodium: 330 mg; Dietary fiber: 0.9 gm.

Orange-Glazed Chicken

SERVINGS: 2 Serving size: ¹⁄₆ of chicken (e.g., ¼ breast plus 1 wing or ½ back, 1 thigh and drumstick)

4–5 lb. Chicken pieces, on bone
or
2–3 lb. Boneless, skinless breasts and thighs
1½ Tbsp. Olive oil
Salt and pepper to taste
1 cup Orange juice, divided in half
1½ tsp. Cornstarch

Brush chicken with olive oil; sprinkle with salt and pepper to taste. Place in 9 x 13 baking pan with ½ cup of the orange juice, and cover with foil. Bake in preheated oven at 375 degrees for 45 minutes, then remove cover to allow chicken to brown.

ORANGE GLAZE: While chicken is baking, mix the rest of the orange juice with the cornstarch; stir until cornstarch is dissolved. Pour into small saucepan and heat over medium to high heat, stirring constantly until boiling and thick. When chicken is done, brush with glaze; return to oven for 5 minutes and serve.

SERVING SUGGESTION: Great with sherried or orange yams and sautéed green beans (see recipes on pgs. 135 and 137).

VARIATIONS: Add mushrooms, celery, peppers, cauliflower, asparagus, or other vegetables to the pan and bake with the chicken.

NUTRITIONAL ANALYSIS FOR ¹⁄₆ RECIPE: Calories: 210; Protein: 23 gm; Carbohydrates: 6 gm; Fat: 10 gm; Saturated fat: 2 gm; Cholesterol: 73 gm; Sodium (without added salt): 70 mg.

DINNER

Stir-Fried Chicken over Rice

SERVINGS: 4 Serving size: ¼ of recipe (½ cup cooked rice plus approx. 1½–2 cups stir-fry mixture)

Mix marinade ingredients together and pour over chicken in a shallow baking pan. Cover and refrigerate while getting other ingredients ready (chicken can marinate for a longer time, if you want to get it ready ahead of time).

Place brown rice and water in saucepan over high heat. Bring to a boil, cover pan tightly, and reduce heat to simmer and cook for 45 to 50 minutes.

Slice onion, carrots, broccoli, and mushrooms into thin pieces. Chop or crush garlic and grate ginger (to save time, buy presliced vegetables and use jarred crushed or chopped garlic, and pregrated ginger).

Heat a heavy, large frying pan or wok over high heat; when pan is hot add ½ of the peanut and sesame oil and all of the garlic and ginger. Stir for 1 minute, until the garlic and ginger has browned. Add the carrots, sauté for 3–5 minutes, then add the onion, broccoli, and mushrooms and sauté for another 5–10 minutes, until the vegetables are just beginning to soften. Remove vegetables from pan; add the other half of the oils. Drain the chicken, but reserve the marinade. Add the chicken to the pan and sauté until cooked through; add the vegetables back to the pan, and sauté together with the chicken for 2–5 minutes. If using frozen vegetables, cook chicken first; add vegetables when chicken is almost done cooking.

¾ cup Brown rice, uncooked
1½ cup Water
1 lb. Chicken breast, boneless, skinless, cut in thin strips

Optional:
Use pork, beef, shrimp, scallops, or firm fish in place of chicken.

Vegetarian option: Use tofu or white beans or garbanzo beans in place of chicken

MARINADE FOR CHICKEN:
¼ cup White wine (e.g., Chablis)
2 Tbsp. Dry sherry
1–3 tsp. Garlic, crushed
1–3 tsp. Ginger, fresh, grated
1 tsp. Prepared mustard
1 dash Black pepper, ground

Optional:
Use ¼ cup white wine vinegar or rice vinegar and 1 Tbsp. brown sugar in place of white wine and sherry

Optional:
Oyster sauce (commercial) 2–4 Tbsp.

Optional:
Plum sauce (commercial) 2–4 Tbsp.

VEGETABLES:

¼–½ medium Onion, thinly sliced

  2 Carrots, thinly sliced

  1 bunch Broccoli, thinly sliced

 10 medium Mushrooms, thinly sliced

Optional:
Vary vegetables—green beans, cauliflower, zucchini, crookneck or summer squash, and bell peppers are all very good in stir-fry. Frozen vegetables can be used to save time.

OTHER INGREDIENTS:

  1 Tbsp. Peanut or canola oil

  1 tsp. Sesame oil

  1 tsp. Garlic, chopped or crushed

1–2 tsp. Ginger, fresh, grated

  2 Tbsp. Cornstarch

  1 cup Low-sodium, fat-free chicken broth

Optional:
¼ cup Cashews, coarsely chopped

Optional:
¼–½ cup Basil, fresh, chopped

Optional:
Add diced, fresh pineapple or thin wedges of fresh tomato and cook for 1–2 minutes right before serving.

Mix the marinade with the chicken broth and cornstarch until the cornstarch is completely dissolved. Add to the pan with the chicken and vegetables, stirring constantly, until the sauce thickens and appears clear. If too thick, add more chicken broth or water.

Add cashews and basil; sauté for another minute or two and serve over the cooked rice (approximately ½ cup of rice and 1–2 cups of stir-fry per person).

SUPER-EASY VERSION:

• Start quick-cooking brown rice in a saucepan.

• Use precut strips of boneless, skinless chicken, and brown in large frying pan with a little oil.

• Add bag of frozen vegetables (broccoli, green beans, or mixed vegetables).

• Mix 1¾ cups low-sodium chicken broth with ¼ cup Teriyaki sauce and 2 Tbsp. cornstarch; stir until smooth. Pour over chicken and vegetables and stir until sauce thickens. Enjoy over brown rice

NUTRIENT ANALYSIS FOR ¼ RECIPE: Calories: 510; Protein: 38 gm; Carbohydrates: 56gm; Fat: 14 gm; Saturated fat: 2.5 gm; Cholesterol: 66 mg; Sodium: 530 mg; Dietary fiber: 7.5 gm (sodium is reduced if oyster and plum sauces are not used; in those cases, increase garlic, ginger, and basil).

Simple Broiled or Grilled Salmon, Halibut, or Cod Fish

SERVINGS: 2   Serving size: approx. 5 oz. cooked fish

Coat broiler pan or barbeque grill with nonstick spray. Mix olive oil, crushed or chopped garlic, lemon juice, and dill weed together in a small bowl. Brush mixture on fish; broil or grill for 10 to 20 minutes (about 10 minutes per inch thickness of fish).

SERVING SUGGESTION: Great with steamed baby red potatoes and tossed green salad.

NUTRITIONAL ANALYSIS FOR ½ RECIPE: Calories: 350 (using Coho salmon); Protein: 36 gm; Carbohydrates: 1.5 gm; Fat: 22 gm; Saturated fat 3.5 gm; Cholesterol 105 mg; Sodium 230 mg (with salt), 83 mg (without salt).

Nonstick cooking spray
¾ lb. Salmon or any other firm fish fillet
1 Tbsp. Olive oil
2 Tbsp. Fresh lemon juice
½ tsp. Dill weed, dried
(if fresh, use 1 tsp.)
⅛ tsp. Salt
⅛ tsp. Pepper

Orange Teriyaki-Flavored Fish

SERVINGS: 3   Serving size: approx. 3½–4 ounces cooked fish

1 **lb. Salmon, halibut, or cod**

SAUCE:

1 **Tbsp. Peanut or canola oil**

Optional:

1 **tsp. Sesame oil**

1–2 **tsp. Garlic, fresh, crushed or minced**

½–1 **tsp. dry Ginger, fresh, grated**

2 **Tbsp. Dry sherry**

1 **Tbsp Soy sauce**

1 **Tbsp. Rice vinegar**

2 **Tbsp. Brown sugar**

¼ **cup Orange juice**

2 **tsp. Cornstarch**

Optional:
Use commercial Teriyaki sauce, mixed with ¼ cup orange juice, to save time.

Start barbeque grill on high heat, then turn down to medium (if using gas); adjust to medium airflow (if using charcoal); or preheat oven to 400 degrees. Heat small saucepan on top of stove; add peanut or canola oil and sesame oil. When oils are hot, add garlic and ginger; sauté until browned. Add sherry, soy sauce, vinegar, and brown sugar. Stir until sugar is dissolved. Mix orange juice with cornstarch, stir until smooth, then add to pan; stir until mixture is thick and clear. Place fish on foil boat for grill or in baking pan for oven. Brush sauce over fish and grill or bake until fish flakes and its inside is opaque when tested with a fork. Be sure to monitor frequently and brush fish with sauce every 5–10 minutes. Try to keep sauce off surface of foil boat or pan, as it will burn quickly.

SERVING SUGGESTION: Place on top of a bed of brown rice with sautéed veggies on the side.

NUTRITIONAL ANALYSIS: Calories: 290 (using halibut); Protein: 32 gm; Carbohydrates: 14 gm; Fat: 10 gm; Saturated fat: 1 gm; Cholesterol: 48 mg; Sodium: 500 mg (sodium can be decreased to 80 mg if no soy sauce is used—1 Tbsp. soy sauce contributes 420 mg sodium per serving).

DINNER

Fish Tacos with Cabbage and Cilantro

SERVINGS: 4

Mix together the cabbage, cilantro, oil, and lime juice and refrigerate. Place fish on a foil boat. Mix garlic and spices with olive oil and brush over fish. Grill or broil until fish flakes (about 10 minutes per inch of thickness).

Heat tortillas on plate in microwave oven for 1–2 minutes, or wrap in foil and heat in 350-degree oven for 15–20 minutes.

Place ¼ of fish in 1 whole grain flour tortilla or 2 corn tortillas, add ¼ of cabbage mixture, garnish with commercial or homemade salsa (see **Mango-Avocado Salsa** recipe in the salad dressings and dips section) and sour cream and/or plain yogurt.

VARIATIONS: Add whole or refried beans in addition to fish; use **Guacamole** in place of sour cream or yogurt (see recipe on page 149); mix mayonnaise and yogurt with commercial salsa and/or chili powder and cumin in place of sour cream or yogurt; use lettuce or spinach in place of cabbage mixture. Be creative!

NUTRITIONAL ANALYSIS FOR TACOS WITH-OUT GARNISHES: Calories: 280; Protein: 25 gm; Carbohydrates: 24 gm; Fat: 9 gm; Saturated fat: 1 gm; Cholesterol: 42 mg; Sodium: 260 mg; Dietary fiber: 3 gm.

1 cup Shredded green and/or red cabbage
¼ cup Fresh cilantro, chopped
1 tsp. Olive oil
1 tsp. Lime juice
1 lb. Firm, white fish (e.g., cod or halibut)
1 Tbsp. Olive oil
2 cloves or 1 tsp. Garlic, crushed
1 tsp. Mild chili powder
½ tsp. Ground cumin
1 tsp. Lime juice
4 Low-fat, whole-grain flour tortillas, burrito size
or
8 Corn tortillas, 6-inch

Pork Chops and Pears or Apples

SERVINGS: 2   Serving size: 1 pork chop and 1 apple or pear

Nonstick cooking spray

2 **Pork chops**
(3-ounce boneless chop, or
4– to 5-ounce bone-in)
**Black pepper, ground
to taste**

**Optional:
Salt to taste**

2 **Large ripe pears
or apples,
cut in half and cored**
1 tsp. **Lemon juice**
2 Tbsp. **Brown sugar**
½–1 tsp. **Cinnamon, ground**
¼ cup **Dry sherry**

Heat oven to 350 degrees. Cut off fat from edges of pork chops. Spray heavy frying pan with non-stick spray and heat over medium-high heat. Place pork chops in frying pan, sprinkle with salt (if desired) and pepper, and cook until browned on both sides. Place pork chops with pears or apples in a 9 x 13 inch baking pan. Sprinkle meat and fruit with lemon juice. Mix brown sugar and cinnamon and sprinkle over meat and fruit; pour sherry over meat and fruit.

Cover with foil and bake at 350 degrees for 20 minutes; remove foil and bake for another 20 minutes, and serve.

VARIATION: Add 1-inch chunks of carrots, yam, or sweet potatoes, cauliflower, onions, and/or celery to pork chops while baking.

SERVING SUGGESTION: Great with baked yams or sweet potatoes and steamed broccoli.

NUTRITIONAL ANALYSIS: Calories: 405; Protein: 21 gm; Carbohydrates: 45 gm; Fat: 14 gm; Saturated fat: 5 gm; Sodium: 46 mg (without added salt); Dietary fiber: 6.6 gm.

Tacos

SERVINGS: 4 Serving size: 1 flour tortilla or 2 corn tortillas

Sauté meat with onions, garlic, and spices. Heat refried beans in a separate pan on stove or in a bowl in microwave. Grate cheese and chop vegetables while meat is cooking. Heat tortillas in microwave or wrap in foil and heat in 350-degree oven.

Assemble taco by placing ¼ beans and ¼ meat mixture in each flour tortilla, or ⅛ of beans and meat in each corn tortilla; top with cheese and then lettuce and tomato. Garnish with fat-free sour cream or plain nonfat yogurt and salsa or picante sauce.

VARIATIONS: Increase amount of onion and bell pepper and add other chopped vegetables to meat mixture to increase number of servings per recipe (you may need to increase garlic and spices for flavor). Use beans without meat for a vegetarian option!

NUTRITIONAL ANALYSIS FOR ¼ RECIPE: Calories: 380; Protein: 24 gm; Carbohydrates: 51 gm; Fat: 11 gm; Saturated fat: 4 gm; Cholesterol: 60 mg; Sodium: 890 mg (sodium can be decreased by using homemade refried beans and reduced-sodium cheese); Dietary fiber: 13 gm.

1 16-oz. can Nonfat refried beans or whole black, pinto, or kidney beans
½ lb. Leanest ground beef
¼ medium Onion, chopped
½–1 tsp. Garlic, chopped or crushed
¼ tsp. Oregano, dried
½ tsp. Cumin, ground
2 tsp. Chili powder

Optional:
½ medium Green, red, or yellow bell pepper, finely diced
1 pinch Ground cardamom and pinch of ground coriander
1 Tbsp. Lime juice
¼ cup Fresh cilantro, chopped

2 oz. Cheddar or jack cheese, shredded
2 cups Romaine or green leaf lettuce, chopped
2 Tomatoes, diced
4 Low-fat, whole-grain flour tortillas, burrito size
   or
8 Corn tortillas, 6-inch
½ cup Nonfat sour cream
½ cup Salsa or picante sauce

Beef and Broccoli Stir-fry

SERVINGS: 4

½ **lb. Lean beef** (e.g., round steak or sirloin steak), **cut in thin slices**

MARINADE:
½ **cup Red wine**

Optional:
Use ¼ cup red wine vinegar and ¼ cup water

¼ **cup Soy sauce**
2 **Tbsp. Brown sugar**
2 **tsp. Garlic, crushed or finely chopped**
2–3 **sprigs Fresh basil,** (about 1/4 cup) **finely chopped**

VEGETABLES:
1 **cup Onion, thinly sliced**
4 **cups Broccoli, fresh, thinly sliced**
or
3 **cups Broccoli, frozen, chopped**

Optional:
1–2 **cups Mushrooms, fresh, sliced or quartered**
1 **Tbsp. Oil (olive, canola, peanut, corn)**
1–2 **tsp. Garlic, crushed or finely chopped**
1–2 **cups Beef broth, low-sodium**
1½ **Tbsp. Cornstarch**

Mix ingredients of marinade together; pour over meat in a shallow pan and refrigerate for an hour to overnight. Heat heavy frying pan and add oil; when oil is hot, add garlic and sauté until browned (about 30 seconds). Remove meat from marinade with slotted spoon to drain off liquid and add to pan; reserve marinade. Sauté for 2–3 minutes and add onion, broccoli, and mushrooms. Sauté for 5–10 minutes, until meat is almost browned and broccoli is just tender-crisp. Mix reserved marinade with 1 cup beef broth and cornstarch, and stir until cornstarch is dissolved. Pour into pan and stir until liquid thickens and clears. Add more broth as needed to get to desired consistency.

SERVING SUGGESTION: Serve over cooked whole-grain noodles, rice, quinoa, couscous, or spelt; or add more beef broth and eat as beef with broccoli soup.

NUTRITIONAL ANALYSIS: Calories: 280; Protein: 30 gm; Carbohydrates: 19 gm; Fat: 7 gm; Saturated Fat: 1 gm; Cholesterol: 44 mg; Sodium: 450 gm; Dietary fiber: 1 gm.

Beef, Chicken, or Pork Fajitas

SERVINGS: 4

Mix meat and vegetables with oil and spices; grill, broil, or stir-fry in heavy frying pan until vegetables are tender-crisp.

Heat beans in microwave or in saucepan with a little water. Place ¼ of the meat and vegetables and beans in 1 flour tortilla or 2 corn tortillas. Garnish with whichever condiments you like, and enjoy!

●

NUTRITIONAL ANALYSIS FOR ¼ RECIPE (using chicken breast and 2 corn tortillas per person): Calories: 365; Protein: 24 gm; Fat: 7 gm; Saturated fat: 1 gm; Cholesterol: 34 mg; Sodium: 212 mg; Dietary fiber: 11 gm (if using beans cooked from dry, with no added salt, subtract 123 mg sodium).

½ **lb. Boneless lean beef, chicken, or pork, thinly sliced**

2 **tsp. Garlic, crushed or finely chopped**

2 **Tbsp. Olive oil**

1 **Tbsp. Chili powder**

1 **tsp. Ground cumin**

1 **tsp. Oregano, dried**
  (if fresh, use 2 tsp.)

⅛ **tsp. Cardamom, ground**

⅛ **tsp. Coriander, ground**

1 **medium Onion, sliced**

½ **of each Green, red, and yellow bell pepper cut in thin strips**

16 **oz. can Black, pinto, red, or kidney beans, drained and rinsed**
  or

1¾ **cups Cooked dry beans**

4 **Low-fat, whole-grain flour tortillas, burrito size**
  or

8 **Corn tortillas, 6-inch**

Condiments (amounts vary to taste):
Salsa, commercial, or Mango-Avocado Salsa **(see recipe on page 149)**
Sour cream, yogurt, or sour cream and yogurt mixture
Avocado slices or guacamole (see Guacamole **recipe on page 149)**

Beef, Chicken, or Pork Peanut Curry over Rice

SERVINGS: 4   Serving size: ¼ recipe (¾ cup rice and about 1½ to 2 cups curry)

1 cup Brown rice

2 cups Water

¾–1 lb. Lean, boneless beef, chicken, or pork, cut in ½- to 1-inch chunks

2 Tbsp. Oil (olive, corn, canola, or peanut)

1 medium Onion, chopped

3 medium Carrots, cut into thin rounds

1 large Bell pepper (red, green, yellow, or orange), cut into 1-inch pieces

2 cups Cauliflower, cut into 1-inch pieces

1 tsp. Cumin, ground

½ tsp. Coriander, ground

½ tsp. Cardamom, ground

or

1 Tbsp. Curry powder (in place of cumin, coriander, and cardamom)

1 tsp. Ginger, fresh

or

½ tsp. Dried ground ginger

⅛ tsp. Dry mustard

1 tsp. Garlic, crushed or chopped

or

½ tsp. Garlic powder

1 16-oz. can Tomatoes, diced, no added salt

1½ cups Low-sodium chicken broth (reserve ¼ cup)

2 Tbsp. Cornstarch

Optional:

¼ cup Raisins

¼ cup Crunchy, natural peanut butter

¼–½ cup Fresh cilantro or basil, chopped

Place rice and water in a saucepan and bring to a boil. Cover, turn heat to very low, and simmer for 45 to 50 minutes, until water is completely absorbed by rice. Prepare the curry while the rice is cooking.

Heat heavy, large saucepan. Add olive oil; when oil is hot, add meat. Sauté meat for 3–4 minutes and add vegetables and spices; sauté until meat is browned and vegetables are slightly soft. Add canned tomatoes and all but ¼ cup chicken broth. Simmer until vegetables are soft. Add raisins. Mix ¼ cup chicken broth with cornstarch and stir until smooth; pour into pan and stir until liquid thickens. Add basil or cilantro, if desired. Serve over rice.

NUTRITIONAL ANALYSIS FOR ¼ RECIPE (using lean pork and optional ingredients, without rice): Calories: 465; Protein: 33 gm; Carbohydrates: 35 gm; Fat: 22 gm; Saturated fat: 5 gm; Cholesterol: 68 mg; Sodium: 215 mg; Dietary fiber: 7 gm.

Raisins account for 30 calories and 7 gm carbohydrate per serving. Peanut butter accounts for 95 calories, 8 gm fat, 5 gm saturated fat, 160 mg sodium, and 4 gm dietary fiber.

NUTRITIONAL ANALYSIS FOR ¾ CUP COOKED BROWN RICE: Calories: 150; Protein: 4 gm; Carbohydrates: 34 gm; Fat: 1.5 gm; Saturated fat: 0; Cholesterol: 0; Sodium: 0; Dietary fiber: 2 gm.

Black Beans and Rice

SERVINGS: 4   Serving size: ¼ recipe (approx. ¾ cup cooked rice and 1 cup bean mixture)

Start cooking rice while preparing beans. Mix brown rice with water and cook on high until boiling, then cover and cook over very low heat for 40 to 45 minutes. Place olive oil in large pan. Add garlic and onion; cook until onion is tender. Add beans. Add chili powder, cumin, oregano, black pepper, and bell pepper; cook for 15 to 30 minutes. Add cilantro and lime juice. Serve 3/4 cup cooked rice topped with 1/4 of the bean mixture topped with grated cheese, lettuce, tomatoes, nonfat sour cream or yogurt, and salsa or picante sauce to taste.

VARIATION: Omit cheese to take out all saturated fat and cholesterol. Cook beans from dry, with no salt, or rinse canned beans with cold water and use fresh salsa or picante sauce to significantly decrease sodium.

NUTRITIONAL ANALYSIS FOR ¼ RECIPE: Calories: 460; Protein: 17 gm; Carbohydrates: 61 gm; Fat: 17 gm; Saturated fat: 8 gm; Cholesterol: 32 mg; Sodium: 720 mg; Dietary fiber: 10 gm.

1 cup Brown rice
2 cups Water
2 cups Black beans (canned and drained, or cooked from dried)
1 Tbsp. Olive oil
1 tsp. Garlic, chopped or crushed
1 medium Onion, chopped
2 tsp. Chili powder
1 tsp. Cumin, ground
1 tsp. Oregano, dried (if fresh, use 2–3 tsp.)
⅛ tsp. Black pepper, ground
1–1½ Bell pepper, chopped (½ each, red, yellow, and green)
2 Tbsp. Lime juice
½ cup Cilantro, fresh, chopped
2 cups Romaine or green leaf lettuce, chopped
2 Tomato, diced
¼ lb. Cheddar cheese, grated
½ cup Nonfat sour cream
½ cup Salsa or picante sauce

Quesadilla for a Quick Meal

SERVINGS: 1

2 Tortillas, corn (6-inch)
1½ cup Nonfat refried beans
2 Tbsp. Canned, diced green chilies

Optional:
2 Tbsp. Medium or sharp cheddar cheese, grated
2 Tbsp. Salsa or picante sauce

Mix green chilies with refried beans and spread half of mixture over each tortilla. Put on a large plate and cook in microwave, on high heat for 1 to 2 minutes or until hot; top with cheese and return to microwave until cheese is melted. Or place quesadillas on cookie sheet and broil in oven for 2 minutes, or until hot; add cheese and return to oven until cheese is melted. Add salsa or picante sauce and enjoy.

OPTIONAL: Top with chopped tomatoes, bell peppers, lettuce, and nonfat sour cream.

VARIATION: Sodium will be greatly reduced if homemade (no salt added) refried beans and fresh salsa rather than jarred are used.

NUTRITIONAL ANALYSIS: Calories: 310; Protein: 12 gm; Carbohydrates: 50 gm; Fat: 7 gm; Saturated fat: 3 gm; Cholesterol: 15 gm; Sodium: 1040 mg; Dietary fiber: 8.3 gm.

Macaroni and Cheese— better than anything in a box!

SERVINGS: 4   Serving size: approx. 2 cups

2 cups Whole wheat macaroni, dry
8 cups Water for cooking macaroni

CHEESE SAUCE:
2 cups Nonfat milk
2 Tbsp. Cornstarch
2 cups Shredded medium or sharp Cheddar or Swiss cheese

Optional seasonings:
3–4 drops Tabasco Sauce
¼ tsp. Dry mustard
⅛ tsp. Ground black pepper

Bring water to a rapid boil; add macaroni and cook for 8–10 minutes and then drain (macaroni can cook while cheese sauce is being prepared). Shred cheese. Mix cold milk with cornstarch and optional seasonings in a heavy saucepan until cornstarch is dissolved. Heat milk mixture over medium to high heat, stirring constantly until mixture comes to a boil and thickens. Add shredded cheese and stir until melted. Mix with cooked macaroni and serve.

SERVING SUGGESTIONS: Great with green salad, cut-up raw or cooked vegetables, and sliced fruit. A sharper tasting cheese gives more cheese flavor with less cheese!

VARIATIONS: Add ¼ cup cashews for crunch and healthy fats. Add 1½ cups finely chopped broccoli, cauliflower, zucchini, and/or onion to the sauce while it is cooking to replace half the macaroni; this will add more vitamins and cut calories by about 65 per serving. Add black, red, kidney, pinto, white, or garbanzo beans or tofu for protein.

NUTRITIONAL ANALYSIS FOR ¼ RECIPE: Calories: 470; Protein: 26 gm; Carbohydrates: 50 gm; Fat: 19.5 gm; Saturated fat: 12 gm; Cholesterol: 62 mg; Sodium: 425 mg; Dietary fiber: 4.4 gm.

Vegetarian Lasagna

SERVINGS: 8   Serving size: 1 lasagna roll

Cook lasagna noodles according to package instructions; drain and rinse to keep from sticking together. Grate mozzarella and cheddar cheeses; mix grated cheeses, spinach, and ½ of the Parmesan cheese with the ricotta. Spoon about 2 cups of the marinara sauce over the bottom of a 9 x 13 inch baking pan. Divide the cheese and spinach mixture into 8 parts; spread ⅛ of mixture on each cooked lasagna noodle and roll up. Place each lasagna roll in the baking pan, seam side down. Pour the rest of the marinara sauce over the lasagna rolls and sprinkle the remainder of the Parmesan cheese over the top. Bake in a preheated oven at 350 degrees for 30 to 45 minutes, until cheese is melted and sauce is bubbling (internal temperature of lasagna rolls should be about 160 degrees). Allow lasagna to rest for 5–10 minutes after removing from oven, before serving.

- ½ package (8 noodles) Whole wheat lasagna noodles
- ½ lb. Low-fat Mozzarella cheese
- ½ lb. Sharp cheddar cheese
- 1 pint Low-fat ricotta cheese
- ½ cup Parmesan cheese, shredded, divided in half
- 10 oz. Frozen, chopped spinach, thawed and drained
- 6 cups or fresh, chopped spinach
- 6–8 cups Vegetarian Marinara sauce (see recipe on p. 151)

NUTRITIONAL ANALYSIS FOR ⅛ RECIPE: Calories: 480; Protein: 30 gm; Carbohydrates: 36 gm; Fat: 22.7 gm; Saturated fat: 23 gm; Cholesterol: 64 mg; Sodium: 655 mg (using vegetarian marinara sauce, made without added salt); Dietary fiber: 7 gm.

VARIATION: Eggplant Parmesan. Use eggplant instead of lasagna noodles and serve crusty whole-grain bread on the side.

DIRECTIONS: Slice eggplant thinly. Place in single layers on cookie sheets and bake for 5 minutes at 400 degrees; turn and bake for another 5 minutes, or until soft.

Layer sauce, eggplant, spinach, and cheese in large baking pan and top with Parmesan cheese. Bake as in lasagna recipe above.

Soups

• • • • • • • • • • • • • •

Lentil Soup

SERVINGS: 8   Serving size: approx. 2 cups

2 cups Lentils, dried
   (no need to presoak)
4 cups Water
4 cups Vegetable broth,
   low sodium
2 Carrots, grated
4 cloves or 2 tsp. Garlic,
   crushed or chopped
1 medium Onion, chopped
1 cup Cauliflower, chopped
28 oz. can Crushed tomatoes
1 tsp. Oregano, dried
1 tsp. Thyme, dried
1 tsp. Rosemary leaves,
   dried (if using fresh herbs,
   use 2-3 tsp. each)

   Optional:
¼ tsp. Dry mustard
1 tsp. Paprika or chili powder
1 tsp. Curry Powder
¼ cup Basil, fresh, chopped
¼ cup Dry sherry
   Salt and pepper to taste

Place lentils, water, and vegetable broth in a large pot; bring to a boil and then simmer for ¾ to 1 hour or until lentils are soft. Chop onion, crush or chop garlic, grate carrot, and chop cauliflower, and add to pot. Add all of the rest of the ingredients and simmer until vegetables are soft (15 to 20 minutes).

•

VARIATION: Sodium is significantly lower if "no added salt" crushed tomatoes and homemade, salt-free vegetable broth are used (see recipe below).

•

NUTRITIONAL ANALYSIS FOR ⅛ RECIPE: Calories: 220; Protein: 14 gm; Carbohydrates: 40 gm; Fat: 1.1 gm; Saturated fat: 0; Sodium: 475 mg; Dietary fiber: 8 gm.

Homemade Vegetable Broth

Place in large pot: 1 medium onion, cut into chunks; 4–5 celery ribs, with leaves, chopped; 2–4 cloves garlic; 2 carrots cut into large pieces; 3–4 peppercorns (optional: turnip, cut into large pieces; any other fresh vegetables that are getting a bit old in your refrigerator). Cover vegetables with water and bring to a boil; simmer until vegetables are very soft. Drain and use broth in any recipe that calls for vegetable broth.

OPTIONAL: Puree the cooked vegetables in blender and use to thicken soup or gravy.

Butternut Squash and Bean Soup

SERVINGS: 6   Serving size: 1 to 1½ cups

Microwave whole butternut squash for 5 minutes to soften and make it easier to cut in half. Cut squash in half and scrape out seeds. Return to microwave for 15–20 minutes until cooked soft.

While squash is cooking, heat large heavy pot; add olive oil and minced garlic, leek, and red bell pepper; sauté until soft. When squash is cooked, scrape out flesh, add to pot, and mash with potato masher (you can also put mixture into a blender and blend until smooth). Add chicken or vegetable broth and beans. Heat thoroughly, add cilantro, salt, and pepper to taste, and serve.

SERVING SUGGESTION: Garnish with nonfat sour cream and/or fresh sprigs of cilantro.

- 1 **medium Butternut squash**
- 1 **Leek, chopped**
- 1 **large Red bell pepper, diced**
- 4 **cloves or 4 tsp. Garlic, minced or crushed**
- 3 **Tbsp. Olive oil**
- ½ **cup Cilantro, fresh, chopped**
- 1 **16-oz. can Garbanzo beans, rinsed and drained**
- 1 **tsp. Cumin, ground**
- 1 **Tbsp. Chili powder**
- ½ **tsp. Dry mustard**
- 1 **tsp. Sage, dried, ground**
- 4 **cups Chicken or vegetable broth, low-sodium**
- **Salt and pepper to taste**

NUTRITIONAL ANALYSIS FOR ⅙ OF RECIPE: Calories: 240; Protein: 7.1 gm, Carbohydrates: 38 gm; Fat: 8 grams; Saturated fat: 1 gm; Sodium: 335 gm (rinsing beans or using beans cooked from dried without added salt reduces sodium); Dietary fiber: 4 gm.

Vegetables and Salads

The Basic Green Salad (simple and delicious)

Mixed lettuces and greens (romaine, green leaf, red leaf, radish greens, spinach, arugula); toss any or all of these together and top with vinaigrette or light creamy dressing.

VARIATIONS FOR SALADS WITH A FLAIR:

WINTER MIX: Add diced oranges, apples, avocado, and/or chopped walnuts (make just enough for one meal; chopped oranges, apples and avocado do not keep well).

MIXED VEGETABLE: Add sliced or diced carrots, cauliflower, radishes, broccoli, cucumber, mushrooms, jicama, tomato, or avocado (for a salad that is going to keep for a few days, wait to add the tomatoes and avocado separately to each serving).

MEAL IN A SALAD: Add to any of the above mixtures:

Drained, rinsed black, pinto, garbanzo, kidney, white, or any other cooked beans and frozen corn or cooked brown rice, quinoa, couscous, or spelt.

Drained, water-packed tuna, any leftover cooked fish, poultry, or meat, and diced, cooked, cold potatoes, yams, or sweet potatoes.

Be creative—come up with your own salad meal!

Homemade Refried Beans

SERVINGS: 8   Serving size: 1/8 of recipe, approx. 1/2 cup

    2 **cups Pinto, red, or black beans, dry**
       Water to soak beans and for cooking

Soak 2 cups dry beans in 6 to 8 cups water overnight. Drain and cover with 6 to 8 cups water; bring to a boil and then simmer for 2½–3 hours (pinto and red beans), 1½–2 hours (black beans), or until very soft. Make sure beans are totally covered with water for entire cooking time. Drain beans, but reserve liquid. Place cooked beans in large, heavy frying pan with about ½ cup of the reserved liquid. Mash beans with potato masher. Use in any recipe that calls for refried beans. Beans can be frozen in small amounts for use in later recipes.

VARIATION: Before adding beans to frying pan, heat 1 tablespoon olive oil in pan and add crushed garlic, chopped onion, diced green chilies, and/or diced bell pepper, and sauté until soft. Season with cumin, chili powder, oregano, and/or other spices depending on what the beans are being used for.

NUTRITIONAL ANALYSIS FOR ⅛ RECIPE: Calories: 125; Protein: 7.7 gm; Carbohydrates: 23 gm; Fat: 0.6 gm; Saturated fat: 0 gm; Sodium: 1 gm; Dietary fiber: 7.7 gm.

Cooked Greens

Spinach, chard, kale, collard, turnip, or beet greens

These can be eaten alone or added to a wide variety of dishes.

Wash greens thoroughly and sauté in a small amount of oil with diced ham (about ¼ ounce per person). Add to sautéed peppers, carrots, cauliflower, or other vegetables. Chop and add to mashed potatoes, soups, stews, chowders, spaghetti sauce, scrambled eggs, and so on. Steam and serve as a "bed" under fish, poultry, meat, or beans. Use your imagination!

Root and Starchy Vegetables

Carrots, white potatoes, sweet potatoes, yams, turnips, winter squash
Mashed vegetables—more than just potatoes!

In a covered pot with a steamer basket, steam white potatoes and/or sweet potatoes, yams, carrots, or other starchy vegetables with chopped cauliflower, broccoli, green beans, peas, zucchini, or other vegetables . . . be creative. When all the vegetables are soft, mash or whip with a little nonfat or low-fat milk and butter or olive oil; season with crushed garlic or garlic powder, chopped basil, and a little salt and pepper.

Roasted Vegetables

Mix higher-calorie, starchy vegetables with lower-calorie vegetables for a delicious, filling side dish.

Preheat oven to 400 degrees. Cut starchy, longer-cooking vegetables (potatoes, sweet potatoes, yams, carrots, and/or winter squash) into 1-inch cubes, place in 9 x 13 inch baking dish, cover, and microwave for 5 to 10 minutes. Add chunks of onion, cauliflower, celery, asparagus, mushrooms . . . whatever veggies you have on hand. Toss with a little homemade or commercial light balsamic vinaigrette (see recipe on page 147) and crushed or chopped garlic, and bake uncovered in oven for 20–30 minutes or until vegetables are tender.

Basic Yam or Sweet Potato

1 large Yam or sweet potato

Bake whole in microwave or 350-degree preheated oven. Poke a few holes with a fork in yams or sweet potatoes to let steam escape. Baking time varies depending on size of yam. Serving size is about 4 ounces, raw weight (a large yam can serve three people). Eat plain or with a little butter, yogurt, or sour cream.

NUTRITIONAL ANALYSIS FOR ¼ LB. RAW WEIGHT OF YAM (will be about ¾ cup cooked): Calories: 135; Protein: 2 gm; Carbohydrates: 32 gm; Fat: 0; Cholesterol: 0; Sodium: 10 mg; Dietary fiber: 5 gm.

Sweet Potatoes with Sherry or White Wine

SERVINGS: 4   Serving size: 1 potato (2 halves)

4 large Sweet potatoes
3 fl. oz. Dry sherry or dry white wine

Cut sweet potatoes in half lengthwise and place in baking pan. Poke two or three holes in each ½ potato with a fork or sharp knife. Pour sherry or wine over sweet potatoes. Cover with foil and bake in 400-degree preheated oven for 30 to 40 minutes, or until soft when pierced with a fork. Or cover with a plate or plastic wrap and cook in microwave for 8–12 minutes or until soft.

SERVING SUGGESTION: These are moist enough to eat without butter! If you would rather not use wine or sherry, try the **Orange Yams and Sweet Potatoes** recipe below.

NUTRITIONAL ANALYSIS FOR ¼ RECIPE: Calories: 135; Protein: 2 gm; Carbohydrates: 27 gm; Sodium: 73 mg; Dietary fiber: 4 gm.

Orange Yams and Sweet Potatoes

SERVINGS: 8

Preheat oven to 375 degrees. Alternate slices of yam and sweet potato in baking pan or large pie pan (alternate colors will look pretty). Mix cornstarch with orange juice and orange peel and pour over yams and potatoes. Cover and bake for 30–40 minutes, until vegetables are soft when pierced with a knife; uncover and allow to bake for another 10 minutes. These can also be baked in microwave until soft and then finished for 10 minutes in oven.

1 lb. **(2 medium) Yams, peeled, sliced into ½-inch rounds**
1 lb. **(3–4 medium) Sweet potatoes, peeled, sliced into ½-inch rounds**
2 **cups Orange juice**
1 **tsp. Orange peel, grated**
1 **Tbsp. Cornstarch**

VARIATIONS: Garnish with thin slices of fresh basil or sprigs of parsley, or add dried cranberries for a tangy, holiday taste.

NUTRITIONAL ANALYSIS FOR ⅛ RECIPE: Calories: 150; Protein: 2 gm; Carbohydrates: 34 gm; Fat: 0; Cholesterol: 0; Sodium: 37 mg; Dietary fiber: 4 gm.

Roasted Yam or Sweet Potato with Meat or Poultry

Add chunks of yam or sweet potato to roasting chicken, beef, or pork (for small roasts, or sliced meats or chicken, add at beginning of roasting time; for larger roasts, add for last hour of roasting time).

Grilled Veggies

Asparagus: break just above tough bottom part of spear and leave whole or cut into 1- to 2-inch pieces

Zucchini: cut in sticks or rounds

Mushrooms: cut off bottoms and leave whole or cut in half

Onions: cut in 1-inch chunks

Amounts of each vegetable depends on individual preference and number of people you want to serve—1 to 2 cups raw vegetables will make about ½ to 1 cup cooked.

For each 4 cups of raw veggies, use 2–3 Tbsp. of **Italian Vinaigrette Salad Dressing** (see recipe on page 147). Brush vinaigrette over vegetables; grill on barbeque in vegetable grilling basket or in foil boat until just tender. (Watch carefully, as these easily burn!)

VARIATION: Bake in oven at 425 degrees until veggies are soft (about 20 to 40 minutes, depending on size of vegetable pieces).

Steamed Veggies

Place any vegetable or combination of vegetables in a steamer, over water. Bring water to a boil and steam until tender-crisp.

Don't have a steamer? Cover the bottom of the pan with water and add vegetables. Bring to a boil and steam the veggies right in the water—keep an eye on the pan and add more water if it gets dry (you want to use as little water as possible without burning your veggies; this will help to keep the vitamins in the veggies and not in the water).

Sautéed Veggies

Cut veggies into small, thin pieces. Green veggies mixed with some sliced orange, red, or yellow peppers look very pretty!

Heat heavy frying pan; add 1 tsp. oil per person. When oil is hot, add ½ tsp. minced or chopped garlic per person. Add 1 cup raw veggies per person and cook, stirring constantly to allow all veggies to be in contact with the bottom of the pan. Whenever pan gets dry, add a couple tablespoons of water. Cook just until veggies are tender-crisp, and then serve.

Eggplant: Eggplant goes well with strong flavors, like those in Asian stir-fries, curries, or Italian sauces and soups. Peel and cube and add to stir-fries, soups, and stews. Slice eggplant and coat with a little olive oil and garlic, and grill. Serve plain or as a sandwich on whole-grain bread.

Fabulous Fruits

Fruits make good snacks, side dishes, desserts, cereal topping ... and so much more.

The best way to eat them is fresh or frozen, and whole. When we make fruit into juice, we throw away the pulp and skin and keep the "sugar water"—juices contain some vitamins and potassium but do not have nearly as many benefits as whole fruits do. Whole fruits can be eaten alone, or pureed, diced, or sliced and mixed with other foods to provide sweetness and lots of nutrients.

Fruit Smoothie

Fresh or frozen fruit: strawberries, oranges, bananas, apples, grapes, peaches, pineapple, and others

Cut fruit in small pieces. Mash or squeeze, blend in blender or with handheld blender; as more liquid is formed, add ice cubes or frozen fruit to make a thick, frosty, and healthy summer drink.

Fruit and Yogurt Smoothie

SERVINGS: 1

½ **cup Plain nonfat yogurt**
½ **cup Frozen fruit (berries, peaches, banana, or other)**

Blend yogurt and fruit in a blender and drink!

NUTRITIONAL ANALYSIS USING FROZEN BLUEBERRIES: Calories: 95; Protein: 6 gm; Carbohydrates: 18 gm; Sodium: 80 mg; Dietary fiber: 2 gm.

Basic Fruit Salad

Mix together *any* cut-up fresh fruits and you have a great salad—no dressing needed! Add fresh fruit to salads made from vegetables, pasta, rice, other grains, or potato. Use your imagination ... fruits are our natural candy!

Citrus Salad

SERVINGS: 4   Serving size: approx. ¾ cup

Mix together fresh oranges, grapefruit, and fresh pineapple. Serve in a small glass dish for a beautiful appetizer. It is a holiday tradition in my family.

NUTRITIONAL ANALYSIS FOR ¼ RECIPE:
Calories: 62; Protein: 1 gm; Carbohydrates: 16 gm; Sodium: 0; Dietary fiber: 2 gm.

1 **large Grapefruit, peeled and sectioned**
1 **large Orange, peeled and cut into 1-inch chunks**
¼ **medium Pineapple, peeled, cored, and cut into 1-inch chunks**

Whole Grains

BROWN RICE: Mix together 2 parts water to 1 part rice, heat to a boil, and cover. Turn stove burner to lowest heat setting and simmer for 45 to 50 minutes, or until all water is absorbed into rice. (Rice contains no gluten.) Cook with chicken, beef, or vegetable broth for added flavor.

RICE PILAF: Sauté rice with mushrooms, onions, garlic, nuts, carrots, celery, and/or other vegetables in a little oil before adding water or broth for an excellent rice pilaf. For extra flair, add golden or black raisins or other dried fruit.

WHOLE WHEAT COUSCOUS: Mix 1½ parts water to 1 part couscous. Bring water to a boil, add couscous, and bring back to a boil. Remove from heat, cover, and let stand for 5 minutes. Use in the same way as rice—it is a great alternative when you are short on time.

Couscous and Black Bean Salad

SERVINGS: 12   **Serving size: approx. ½ cup**

½ cup Dry, whole wheat couscous
¾ cup Water
1 16-oz. can Black beans, rinsed and drained
1 cup Frozen corn
½ medium Bell pepper (red, green, yellow, and/or orange), diced
1 Tbsp. Onion, finely chopped
1 medium Tomato, diced

Optional:
1 stalk Celery, diced
½ Cucumber, diced
1 tsp. Garlic, crushed
1–2 Tbsp. Lime juice
¼–½ cup Fresh cilantro, chopped
1–2 tsp. Chili powder
½–1 tsp. Ground cumin
1 pinch Salt
1 Tbsp. Olive oil

Add ½ cup couscous to ¾ cup boiling water. Cover, remove from heat, and let stand for 5 minutes. Put into mixing bowl and fluff with a fork. Add frozen corn to couscous (this will cool couscous and thaw corn). Add the rest of the ingredients and mix well. Chill in refrigerator until serving time. Ingredients can all be varied to individual tastes.

VARIATIONS: Use cooked brown rice, bulgur, or quinoa or an extra 1½ cups corn in place of couscous.

FAST VERSION: Combine couscous or other grain, black beans, and corn as above; in place of other ingredients, add 1 cup mild to medium picante sauce or salsa; add cilantro and lime juice as desired.

NUTRITIONAL ANALYSIS FOR 1/12 OF RECIPE: Calories: 92; Protein: 4 gm; Carbohydrates: 17 gm; Fat: 2 gm; Saturated fat: 0; Sodium: 142 mg; Dietary fiber: 4 gm.

CORN: It's a grain! Use fresh corn on the cob or frozen corn for a tasty whole grain. Add chopped onion or red or green pepper for some flair.

QUINOA: Another rice substitute; this is a high-protein grain that is easy to prepare and definitely underused. Mix 1¾ parts water or broth to 1 part quinoa, bring to a boil, turn heat to low, and cook for 15 minutes. (Contains no gluten.)

BARLEY: Place 1 cup "hulled" barley in 3 cups water and soak for 8 hours or overnight. Cook in same liquid for 1–1½ hours, or until soft. Add uncooked barley plus water to soups and stews that require long cooking times for a great whole-grain addition.

BULGUR: Made from cracked wheat, bulgur cooks in about 20 minutes. Mix 2 parts water to 1 part bulgur and simmer, covered, until liquid is all absorbed.

SPELT: Place 1 cup spelt berries in a large bowl; cover with water and soak for 8 hours or overnight. Drain berries, put in a pan with 3 cups boiling water or broth. Cover, reduce heat, and simmer for 1 hour. (If spelt is not soaked first, simmer for 1½ hours.) Use as a hot cereal, in salads, baked goods, soups, stews, and casseroles. Cook large amounts at one time and freeze for later use.

WHOLE-GRAIN PASTA: Whole wheat and multigrain pastas are easy to find these days. Cook them in the same way you cook white pasta and enjoy a much healthier carbohydrate. (Brown rice pastas are available for people with gluten intolerance.)

OATS: Great when cooked as oatmeal, raw, mixed with fruit and/or yogurt, or cooked into muffins, pancakes, waffles, and so on. (Oats are gluten-free, if processed in a plant with no other gluten-containing products.)

READY-TO-EAT CEREALS: Look for a whole grain or whole grain flour as the first ingredient, and for a minimum of 3 gm fiber for every 100 calories of cereal (if the package says 4 grams of fiber per serving, but a serving contains 200 calories, it is not a very high-fiber cereal!). Some so-called healthy cereals contain very little whole grain or fiber—read the labels!

100% WHOLE-GRAIN BREADS: Look for whole grain flour to be the first ingredient (wheat flour is not whole grain unless the label says "whole wheat flour") and for at least 2 gm fiber per slice.

Super Snacks

● ● ● ● ● ● ● ● ● ● ● ● ●

FRESH FRUIT ALL BY ITSELF: This is the original fast food. Cut fruit in pieces for younger kids—a couple of slices, a quarter to a half of an apple, banana, or orange, is fine for a preschooler to an eight-year-old; a whole fruit works for an older child.

FRUIT AND MILK SHAKE—NO SUGAR NEEDED: Put ½ to 1 cup frozen fruit (berries, peaches, ripe banana) into blender, add ½ to 1 cup nonfat or 1% milk, blend, and pour into a glass for an extremely healthy and delicious milk shake.

VEGGIES AND DIP: Keep veggies washed and cut up, ready to eat, in a container in the refrigerator—carrots, celery, cauliflower, cucumber, broccoli . . . tomatoes actually keep better out of the refrigerator. Kids love small grape-size and cherry tomatoes. (See page 148 for dip recipes.)

LEFTOVER SOUP OR CASSEROLE: If your child is very hungry and dinner is a couple of hours away, fill him up with something nourishing and filling, rather than lots of low-nutrient, "snacky" foods.

NUTS, DRY CEREAL, AND DRIED FRUIT: A healthy snack for a hungry child is as easy as combining ¼ cup plain Cheerios or puffed kamut with 2 Tbsp. raisins and 8–10 unsalted almonds. Serve in a small dish or sandwich bag for a snack-on-the-go.

WHOLE-GRAIN CEREAL WITH FRUIT AND MILK: There's nothing wrong with a re-do of breakfast for a snack, and it's far more nutritious than a many of the "snack foods" out there!

WHOLE-GRAIN TOAST OR ENGLISH MUFFIN: Cover with peanut or almond butter and jam or honey.

QUICK QUESADILLA: Spread mashed beans or refried beans on a corn tortilla, add a little cheese, and broil or microwave until hot. Cut into fourths to serve two or three preschoolers or one older child. Make it fancy by adding peppers, tomato, or other vegetables.

Popcorn, the Old-Fashioned Way

SERVINGS: 4   Serving size: 4–6½ cup

Heat large heavy pan or popcorn popper. Add oil and 3–4 kernels popcorn; when that pops, add the rest of the popcorn. If using a pan, move it back and forth on the burner while popcorn is popping to prevent burning. When popping stops, remove pan from heat or turn off popper and pour popcorn into a paper bag or large bowl. Melt butter in microwave and pour over popcorn and shake or stir to distribute evenly; add salt to taste. Store leftovers in a covered container.

¾ cup **Popcorn kernels (unpopped)**
1 Tbsp. **Canola oil**

Optional:
1 Tbsp. **Butter**
Salt to taste

NUTRITIONAL ANALYSIS FOR ¼ RECIPE: Calories: 175; Protein: 4 gm; Carbohydrates: 29 gm; Fat: 8 gm; Saturated fat: 0.3 gm; Cholesterol: <0.5 mg; Sodium: 29 gm (no added salt); Dietary fiber: 6 gm. Without butter: 150 calories; 4 gm fat; 0 gm saturated fat and cholesterol; and 0 gm sodium (no added salt).

NOTE: *Popcorn is not suitable for children under 2–3 years due to risk of choking.*

Desserts

• • • • • • • • • • • • • •

Ice Cream Sundae

SERVINGS: 1

½ cup Ice cream, any flavor
¼ cup Berries, fresh or
  frozen (peaches,
  nectarines, bananas . . .)
1 Tbsp. Chocolate syrup

Place ice cream in very small dish or teacup and arrange fruit over the top—the idea is to make it pretty. Drizzle chocolate syrup over the top of the fruit and ice cream and enjoy.

NUTRITIONAL ANALYSIS: Calories: 215; Protein: 4 gm; Carbohydrates: 30 gm; Fat: 9 gm; Saturated fat: 5 gm; Cholesterol: 25 gm; Sodium: 43 mg; Dietary fiber: 1 gm.

Sautéed Apples and Cinnamon over Yogurt

SERVINGS: 4

1 large (8 oz.) Apple,
  cored, cut in half and
  thinly sliced
1 Tbsp. Butter
1 Tbsp. Brown sugar
½–1 tsp. Cinnamon
2 cups Nonfat plain
  yogurt

Heat frying pan and add butter. When butter is melted, add apples and brown sugar. Sauté until apples are soft; add cinnamon. Divide into fourths and serve over ½ cup plain nonfat yogurt in a small dessert dish or teacup. Apple mixture will be sweet enough to go very well with tartness of plain yogurt.

NUTRITIONAL ANALYSIS FOR ¼ RECIPE: Calories: 125; Protein: 6 gm; Carbohydrates: 20 gm; Fat: 3 gm; Saturated fat: <0.5 gm; Cholesterol: 3 mg; Sodium: 104 mg; Dietary fiber: 2 gm.

Baked Apples

SERVINGS: 1

Preheat oven to 375 degrees. Core whole apples and peel off top ¼ of skin. Use fingers or a butter knife to coat peeled part of apple and inside of core hole with butter. Mix sugar and cinnamon together and sprinkle into core and on peeled part of apple. If desired, put raisins in core of apple.

Place apple in a baking pan, cover, and bake at 375 degrees for ½–¾ hour, until soft when poked with a fork. Take cover off and bake for another 5–10 minutes, or until top is slightly browned. Allow apple to cool for 15–30 minutes before eating.

1 Apple, tart (Granny Smith or Gravenstein are great, but any variety will do)
1 tsp. Butter
2 tsp. Brown sugar
¼ tsp. Cinnamon, ground

Optional:
1 Tbsp. Raisins

NUTRITIONAL ANALYSIS (without raisins): Calories: 137; Protein: 1 gm; Carbohydrates: 27 gm; Fat: 4 gm; Saturated fat: 0; Cholesterol: 0; Sodium: 43 mg; Dietary fiber: 3.5 gm. (Raisins contribute 33 calories, 7.75 gm carbohydrates, and 0.5 gm dietary fiber.)

Broiled Canned Peaches, Apricots, or Pears

Drain peach, apricot, or pear halves that have been canned in light syrup or juice. Place 2 halves per person on a cookie sheet or baking pan. Sprinkle with cinnamon. Broil for 3–5 minutes (check frequently to make sure they do not burn). Serve as is or with yogurt, frozen yogurt, or ice cream.

NUTRITIONAL ANALYSIS: Calories: 85–100; Protein: 0; Fat: 0; Cholesterol: 0; Sodium: 12 mg; Dietary fiber: 1 gm.

Fruit Pudding and Granola Parfaits

SERVINGS: 6

1 small package Vanilla
pudding mix (not instant)
¾ cup Granola (look for
lowest sugar and fat)
1½ cups Frozen or fresh fruit
(peaches, berries, bananas)

Cook pudding according to package instructions, using nonfat or 1% milk. Allow to cool in refrigerator for 10–20 minutes. Use 6 clear glass dessert dishes, parfait cups, or small drinking glasses. Layer pudding, granola, and fruit in each glass (use about ⅓ cup pudding, 2 Tbsp. granola, and ¼ cup fruit for each serving).

VARIATION: Mix together 1 part flavored vanilla yogurt and 1 part plain nonfat yogurt. Layer yogurt, fruit, and granola in a dessert dish, parfait cup, or small drinking glass.

NUTRITIONAL ANALYSIS FOR ⅙ RECIPE: Calories: 140; Protein: 5 gm; Carbohydrates: 30 gm; Fat: 1 gm; Saturated fat: 0; Cholesterol: 2 mg; Sodium: 136 mg; Dietary fiber: 2 gm.

Refreshing Fruit Slushy

SERVINGS: 2

1 cup Fresh fruit, chopped
(berries, peaches,
pear, melon, mango,
pineapple, orange, banana)

Frozen fruit, any kind
(freeze overripe bananas
for use in slushies—peel
bananas and put in plastic
container or freezer bag
and freeze)

Place fresh fruit in blender, or use hand-held immersion blender, and blend until liquefied. Add frozen fruit and continue to blend. Result will be a thick slushy that you can eat with a spoon or drink with a straw

NUTRITIONAL ANALYSIS FOR ½ RECIPE USING BANANA AND ORANGE (other fruits may be slightly lower in calories and carbohydrates): Calories: 110; Protein: 2 gm; Carbohydrates: 28 gm; Fat: 1 gm; Saturated fat: 0; Cholesterol: 0; Sodium: 1 mg; Dietary fiber 4 gm.

Salad Dressings and Dips

● ● ● ● ● ● ● ● ● ● ● ● ● ●

Italian Vinaigrette Salad Dressing

Serving size: 1 Tbsp.

Mix everything but oil together in a blender and blend until smooth (mustard will work as an "emulsifier" and keep all oil and vinegar from separating). Add oil and mix before serving.

●

NUTRITIONAL ANALYSIS FOR 1 TBSP. SALAD DRESSING: Calories: 35 to 65 (depending on amount of oil used); Fat: 4 to 7 gm (depending on amount of oil used); Sodium: 5 mg.

½ cup Balsamic, cider, or
    red wine vinegar
2 Tbsp. Water
½ tsp. Italian seasoning
⅛ tsp. Garlic powder
⅛ tsp. Onion powder
⅛–¼ tsp. Sugar
1 pinch Ground black
    pepper
½ tsp. Dijon or yellow
    mustard
¼–½ cup Olive or canola oil

Asian Salad Dressing

Serving size: 1 Tbsp.

Mix everything but oil together in a jar or salad dressing cruet and shake well. Add oil and shake before serving.

●

NUTRITIONAL ANALYSIS FOR 1 TBSP. SALAD DRESSING: Calories: 48 to 66 (depending on amount of sugar and oil); Fat: 5 to 7 gm (depending on amount of oil); Sodium: 53 mg.

½ cup Rice vinegar
⅛ tsp. Garlic powder
⅛ tsp. Ground ginger powder
⅛–¼ tsp. Sugar
½ tsp. Soy or tamari sauce
¼ tsp. Sesame oil
¼–½ cup Peanut oil

Low-Calorie Thousand Island Dressing

Serving size: 1 Tbsp.

¼ cup Low-fat mayonnaise
¼ cup Plain nonfat yogurt
¼ cup Ketchup (vary amount to get desired flavor)
2 Tbsp. Sweet pickle relish (vary amount to get desired flavor)

Optional:
⅛ tsp. Dry mustard and a few drops lemon juice

Mix all ingredients together until uniform.

VARIATION: Lower sodium to 48 mg per Tbsp. by substituting 3 Tbsp. tomato paste, 1 tsp. brown sugar, and 1 Tbsp. cider vinegar for ketchup.

NUTRITIONAL ANALYSIS FOR 1 TBSP. SALAD DRESSING: Calories: 18; Fat: 1 gm; Sodium: 94 mg.

Creamy Salad Dressing or Dip

Serving size: 1 Tbsp.

½ cup Plain nonfat yogurt,
½ cup Cottage cheese, low-fat, 1%
½ tsp. Onion powder
½ tsp. Garlic powder
¼ tsp. Dill weed, dried
Black pepper to taste

Put all ingredients in blender, or use hand-held blender, and blend until smooth.

VARIATIONS: Blend in chili powder and cumin in place of dill weed for "South of the Border" flavor. Blend in curry powder in place of dill weed for a Middle Eastern flavor.

NUTRITIONAL ANALYSIS FOR 1 TBSP. DIP: Calories: 9; Protein: 1 gm; Sodium: 33 mg.

Guacamole

Serving size: 2 Tbsp.

Mash together with fork until fairly smooth.

VARIATION: Use 5 Tbsp. prepared salsa in place of tomato, garlic, and onion. (This will be higher in sodium, depending on the sodium content of the salsa used.)

NUTRITIONAL ANALYSIS FOR 2 TBSP. DIP:
Calories: 45; Protein: 1 gm; Fat: 4 gm; Sodium: 7 mg.

- 1 medium Avocado, mashed
- ¼ cup Plain nonfat yogurt
- ½ tsp. Garlic, crushed, fresh or jarred
  or
- ¼ tsp. Garlic powder
- ¼ cup Tomato, finely diced
- 1 Tbsp. Onion, finely minced
  or
- ½ tsp. Onion powder
- 1 tsp. Chili powder
- ½ tsp. Ground cumin
- 1 tsp. Lime juice

Mango-Avocado Salsa

SERVINGS: 4

Mix together. Vary ingredients as desired for personal preference.

NUTRITIONAL ANALYSIS FOR ¼ RECIPE:
Calories: 130; Protein: 2 gm; Carbohydrates: 16 gm; Fat: 8 gm; Saturated fat: 1 gm; Cholesterol: 0; Sodium: 13 mg; Dietary fiber: 5 gm.

- 1 medium Mango, fresh, peeled and diced
- 1 small Avocado, fresh, peeled and diced
- 1 small Tomato, diced
- ½ cup Red, yellow, or green bell pepper, chopped
- 2 Tbsp. Onion (red, yellow, or white), finely chopped
- 2 cloves or 1 tsp. Garlic, finely chopped or crushed
- ¼ cup Fresh cilantro, chopped
- 2 tsp. Lime juice
- 1 tsp. Mild chili powder
- ½ tsp. Ground cumin

Basic Sauces, Marinades, and Rubs

● ● ● ● ● ● ● ● ● ● ● ● ●

Marinara Sauce with Low-fat Chicken or Turkey Italian Sausage

SERVINGS: 8   Serving size: ⅛ of recipe, approx. 1½ cups per serving

1 lb. **Turkey or chicken Italian sausage, or very lean ground meat**
4 **cloves or 4 tsp. Garlic, crushed or chopped**
1–2 **tsp. each Herbs, dried: marjoram, rosemary, thyme, oregano**
(if fresh, use 1-2 Tbsp. each)
⅛–¼ **cup Basil, fresh, chopped**
1–2 **Bay leaves**
2 **cups Mushrooms, sliced**
1 **small Onion, chopped**
12 **oz. can Tomato paste**
(no added salt)
29 **oz. can Tomatoes, chopped or tomato puree**
(no added salt)

Optional:
1 **cup Red wine** (e.g., Burgundy)
Water as desired to thin to desired consistency

Brown sausage or ground meat with onions, garlic, herbs, mushrooms, and optional vegetables. Add wine, tomatoes or tomato puree, and tomato paste. Stir until paste is well distributed in sauce; add water to thin to desired consistency. Bring to a boil, turn heat down, and simmer for 30–60 minutes.

●

OPTIONAL: Chopped red, yellow, and/or green bell pepper, grated zucchini, grated carrot, finely chopped broccoli or cauliflower (adds flavor and nutrition without increasing calories). If optional vegetables are added, you can get more servings out of one recipe.

●

OPTIONAL: Use any type of cooked beans in place of meat; when served over pasta or grain, you have a complete protein.

●

NUTRITIONAL ANALYSIS FOR ⅛ RECIPE WITHOUT OPTIONAL VEGETABLES: Calories: 200; Protein: 15 gm; Carbohydrates: 21 gm; Fat: 5 gm; Saturated fat: 1.2 gm; Cholesterol: 43 mg; Dietary fiber: 4.5 gm; Sodium: 410 mg (sodium will be much less if ground meat rather than sausage is used).

Vegetarian Marinara Sauce with Fresh Herbs

SERVINGS: 8   Serving size: 1½ to 2 cups

Use for any recipe that calls for marinara or tomato-based sauce.

Heat heavy pot. Add olive oil and rotate pan so that the bottom is totally covered. Add garlic and onion and sauté until soft; then add grated and chopped vegetables and mushrooms and herbs; continue to sauté until these are soft. Add wine, tomato paste, diced or crushed tomatoes, and water, and simmer for 30–45 minutes. Taste and add salt and pepper and other seasonings as desired.

●

NUTRITIONAL ANALYSIS FOR ⅛ OF RECIPE WITHOUT ADDED SALT: Calories: 200; Protein: 5.3 gm; Carbohydrates: 26 gm; Fat: 7.8 gm; Saturated fat: 1.1 gm; Cholesterol: 0; Sodium: 100 mg; Dietary fiber: 6 gm.

4   Tbsp. Olive oil
4   cloves or 4 tsp. Garlic, chopped or crushed
1   small Onion, finely chopped
1   medium Zucchini, grated
1   medium Carrot, grated
1   medium Green bell pepper, finely chopped
1   medium Red bell pepper, finely chopped
1   medium Yellow bell pepper, finely chopped
2   cups Mushrooms, sliced
1   Tbsp. Fresh marjoram
1   Tbsp. Fresh rosemary
1   Tbsp. Fresh thyme
    (if using dried marjoram, rosemary, and thyme, use 1 tsp.)
¼   cup Fresh basil, chopped
    (if using dried basil, use 1 Tbsp.)
1–2   Bay leaves

Optional:
1   cup Burgundy or other red wine

12   oz. can Tomato paste, no added salt
29   oz. can Diced or crushed tomatoes, no added salt
     Water to thin to desired consistency

Optional:
Salt and pepper to taste; dry mustard, chili powder, and/or cayenne pepper
(start with approx. ⅛ tsp. and increase to taste)

White Sauce

1 cup Nonfat or 1% milk
1 Tbsp. Cornstarch
Salt and pepper to taste

Optional:
1 pinch Dry mustard
2–3 drops Tabasco sauce

Stir cold milk and cornstarch together with a fork or wire whip until starch is totally dissolved. Pour in a saucepan. Cook over medium to high heat, stirring constantly until boiling and thick (about 5–7 minutes).

Use to make creamed vegetables or meat; as gravy base (add meat drippings or broth for flavor); as soup base (add vegetable, chicken, or beef broth plus vegetables and/ or leftover meat for a quick cream soup); and as a cheese sauce base (add 1 cup grated cheese per cup of milk). Vary amount of cornstarch for the desired thickness.

NUTRITIONAL ANALYSIS FOR WHOLE RECIPE: Calories: 120; Protein: 9 gm; Carbohydrates: 20 gm; Fat: 0; Cholesterol: 5 mg; Sodium: 135 mg; Dietary fiber: 0.

Sweet-and-Sour Beef Marinade

½ cup Dry red wine (e.g., Burgundy)
2–3 Tbsp. Soy sauce
2–3 Tbsp. Brown sugar
1 Tbsp. Oil (canola or peanut)

Optional:
2–3 tsp. Crushed or minced garlic
2-3 tsp. Chopped fresh basil or cilantro
1 tsp. Grated fresh ginger

Savory Beef Marinade

1 cup **Dry red wine**
(e.g., Burgundy)

1 Tbsp. **Italian seasoning**
or

1 Tbsp. **each Chopped**
fresh herbs (basil, rosemary,
oregano, thyme, marjoram)

1 Tbsp. **Crushed or minced**
garlic

1 Tbsp. **Onion flakes**

Optional:

1 tsp. **Dijon mustard**
Salt and pepper to taste

1–2 Tbsp. **Olive oil**

Orange Chicken Marinade

¾ cup **Orange juice**
(fresh or frozen)

1 Tbsp. **Soy sauce**

1–2 tsp. **Garlic, crushed or**
minced

½–1 tsp. **Ginger, grated, fresh**

1–2 Tbsp. **Oil** (canola or peanut)

Optional:

1 tsp. **Orange rind, finely**
grated
Fresh basil or cilantro,
chopped
Dry sherry

Savory Chicken Marinade

1 cup **Dry white wine** (e.g., Chablis)
1 Tbsp. **Italian seasoning**
   or
1 Tbsp. each **Fresh herbs, chopped**
   (basil, oregano, rosemary, thyme, marjoram)
2–4 tsp. **Garlic, crushed or minced**

Optional:
2 tsp. **Onion flakes, dried**
   or
2 Tbsp. **Onion, fresh, minced**
1 Tbsp. **Olive oil**
1 tsp. **Dijon mustard**

Gravy/Sauce for Meat, Poultry, or Stir-fry

½–1 cup **Marinade reserved after marinating meat**
(use any of above recipes for marinade)
1 cup **Beef or chicken broth**
1½ Tbsp. **Cornstarch**

Mix together with fork or wire whip until all lumps are dissolved, add ½–1 cup reserved marinade, and cook over medium-high heat, stirring constantly until boiling and thickened.

Rubs for Any Meat, Poultry, Fish, or Vegetables

GENERAL DIRECTIONS FOR ALL RUBS: Rub the mixture all over meat before grilling, baking, or broiling, or toss with vegetables before sautéing or roasting. If cooking chicken with the skin on, put rub underneath chicken skin. Double or triple recipe as needed to thoroughly coat meat or vegetables.

Vary the flavors of any of these marinades or sauces by adding brown or white sugar; honey; fruit juice; grated lemon, lime, or orange rind; Dijon, brown, yellow, or other mustards; horseradish; different types of wine (e.g., dry sherry or marsala), beer, or other liquors. You can mix oil with whatever herbs, spices, or juices smell good to you and then brush on any meat, poultry, fish, or vegetable.

Herb and Garlic Rub

2 Tbsp. Olive oil
1 tsp. each Herbs, dried
(rosemary, thyme, oregano, basil)
(if fresh, use 1 Tbsp. each)
2-3 tsp. Garlic, crushed or minced
2 tsp. Onion flakes, dried
(if fresh, use 2 Tbsp. minced)
1 pinch Black pepper

Optional:
1 pinch Salt

Ginger Garlic Rub

2 Tbsp. Olive oil or peanut oil
2-3 tsp. Garlic, crushed or minced
1-2 tsp. Ginger, fresh, grated
1 tsp. Sugar
1 Tbsp. Soy sauce

Lemon Garlic Rub

2 Tbsp. Olive oil
2-3 tsp. Garlic, crushed or minced
1 Tbsp. Lemon juice
¼ tsp. Lemon peel, finely grated

Optional:
Salt and pepper to taste
Fresh or dried dill weed or parsley
to taste

Mustard Dill Rub

- **1 Tbsp. Dijon mustard**
- **2 Tbsp. Olive oil**
- **1 tsp. Lemon juice**
- **½ tsp. Dill weed, fresh**
  (if dried, use ¼ tsp.)

Honey Mustard Curry Rub

- **1 Tbsp. Dijon mustard**
- **1 Tbsp. Honey**
- **¼ cup Orange juice**
- **½ tsp. Ginger, fresh, grated**
- **1 tsp. Curry powder**

Raise Your Nutritional IQ

A Detailed Look
at the Five Food Groups

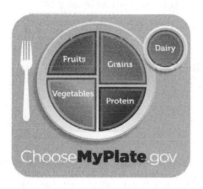

WHAT DOES A "HEALTHY" DIET LOOK LIKE?

This section gives you an overview of what all of us need to eat to meet our nutritional needs. It outlines the different food groups and gives the positives and negatives of each. For more information, go to www.choosemyplate.gov.

Goals for a healthy diet:

3–4 servings/day milk or other dairy products

1 serving = 1 cup milk, 1½ oz. cheese, 6 oz. yogurt

2–3 servings protein foods (meat/beans/nuts/eggs)

1 serving = 3 oz. meat (size of a deck of cards), ½ cup beans, 2 eggs, 2 tablespoons peanut butter, ¼ cup nuts

5 servings vegetables

1 serving = ½ cup cooked, 1 cup raw

2 servings fruit

1 serving = 1 piece fresh fruit (e.g., 1 apple, 1 medium banana), 1 cup cut-up fresh fruit, ½ cup canned fruit, ¼ cup dried fruit, ½ cup fruit juice

6–9 servings grains

(More if very active!) Aim for at least half to be whole grains.

1 serving = 1 small slice bread, ¼ bagel or ½ English muffin, ½ cup cooked rice or pasta, 1 tortilla, 1 small roll, ⅔ cup hot cereal, 1 oz. dry cereal

Details of each food group

Dairy—milk and foods made from milk—important nutrients:

- Calcium: Important for building and maintaining bones.
- Vitamin D: Important for bone development and our immune systems.
- Protein: Important for growth and development in children, maintaining healthy cells, and healing wounds.
- Riboflavin (Vitamin B2): Helps metabolize energy and protein.
- Vitamin A: Important for vision, our immune system, and reproduction.

Dairy—less healthy aspects:

- Saturated fat and cholesterol: May contribute to heart disease (full-fat milks, yogurts, cheeses, cream, ice cream)

Recommendations:

- Choose nonfat or low-fat milk and yogurt for main sources of dairy products.
- Use cheeses (even low-fat cheeses), cream, and full-fat dairy products sparingly.
- Try nonfat or low-fat soy, almond, or rice milk (high-calcium alternatives to cow or goat milk).

Protein foods—meat, poultry, fish, eggs, legumes (beans, peas, lentils, and peanuts), and tree nuts—important nutrients:

- Iron: Iron is an essential part of red blood cells, which carry oxygen to all the cells of our bodies.

- B-vitamins: Help with metabolism of the energy we eat and maintain healthy cells.
    - ○ Niacin: Meats, poultry, and fish
    - ○ Riboflavin: Meats, poultry, and fish
    - ○ Pantothenic acid: Chicken, beef, egg yolk, organ meats
    - ○ Thiamin: Pork
    - ○ Vitamin B12: All animal products—meat, poultry, fish, eggs, milk, and other dairy products.
    - ○ Folic acid: Legumes
- Vitamin A: (see dairy section) Fish and organ meats.
- Vitamin D: (see dairy section) Fish and sea mammals.
- Zinc: Meats, poultry, and fish. Zinc is critical for growth and development, involved in many metabolic processes in our bodies.
- Heart-healthy fats: Fish and shellfish, nuts.

Protein foods—less healthy aspects:

- Saturated fat and cholesterol: High-fat meats and poultry, egg yolk, cheese.
- Sodium: Processed meats and poultry.

Recommendations:

- Eat more legumes, fish, and very low-fat meats (skinless chicken, grass-fed beef, game, and lean pork).
- Avoid high-fat meats, processed meats (hot dogs, bologna, bacon, sausage, deli meats).
- Limit red meats.

Vegetables and fruits—important nutrients:

- Vitamin A: Dark yellow/orange and dark leafy green vegetables.
- Vitamin C: Broccoli, potatoes, tomatoes, cabbage, citrus fruits, kiwi, papaya, mango.
- Folic acid: Dark green leafy vegetables, broccoli, oranges.
- Vitamin K: Dark green leafy vegetables.
- Potassium: Potatoes, sweet potatoes, tomatoes, dark green leafy vegetables,

bananas, mangos, oranges, peaches, apricots . . . all vegetables and fruits contain some potassium.

- Magnesium: Dark green vegetables.
- Fiber: All fruits and vegetables. Helps maintain intestinal health, prevents diverticulitis, helps lower blood cholesterol.

Recommendations:

- Eating vegetables helps prevent heart disease and possibly some cancers. Taking the nutrients or antioxidants found in vegetables in a pill form does not have the same effect.

Grains—important nutrients:

- Fiber: Whole grains.
- B vitamins: Whole grains and enriched refined (white) grains and ready-to-eat cereals.
- Iron: Whole grains and enriched refined grains and ready-to-eat cereals.
- Zinc: Whole grains.

Grains—less healthy aspects:

- Low nutritional value: Refined grains (white flour, white rice, white pasta, cereals made from refined grains) give calories with little nutritional value, other than added vitamins and iron.

Recommendations:

- Eat more whole grains: whole-grain pasta, brown rice, 100 percent whole wheat breads, rolls and tortillas, quinoa, corn, whole wheat couscous.
- Limit refined flour and grain products: white breads, rolls, tortillas, ready-to-eat cereals with less than 3 gm fiber per 100 calories, white rice, white pasta, sweets made with white flour.

Carbohydrates, Fat, and Protein

A Detailed Look
at the Major Components of Foods

F OODS ARE MADE UP OF CARBOHYDRATES, PROTEIN, AND FAT
and we need a balance of all three. These nutrients come in many
different forms, some healthier than others. This appendix gives you
a basic understanding of each food component and takes the mystery
out of ingredients such as "high fructose corn syrup" and "trans fats."

● ● ● ● ● ● ● ● ● ● ● ● ● ●

Carbohydrates contain about 4 calories per gram (to put this into
perspective, table sugar has about 4 grams of carbohydrate and 16 calories
per teaspoon). We can divide carbohydrates into three categories—complex,
simple, and fiber.

Complex carbohydrates are what we commonly think of as starch.
They do not taste sweet, but they break down into sugar in our intestines
before they are absorbed into our bloodstream. Starches are made from
long strings of glucose molecules all attached to each other. We want most of
our carbohydrates to be complex; because these take longer to absorb than
simple carbohydrates do, they raise our blood sugar more slowly and keep
us feeling satisfied for longer than the same amount of calories in simple
carbohydrates.

Simple carbohydrates are what we think of as sugar—they vary in sweetness. Milk sugar, lactose, is made from the two molecules glucose and galactose. These are stuck together and give a little sweet taste to milk; lactose is not nearly as sweet-tasting as glucose by itself. Lactose is separated into glucose and galactose in our small intestine before it is absorbed. (People who do not have the enzyme necessary to break lactose apart are "lactose intolerant.")

Table sugar, made from sugar cane or sugar beets, is sucrose; it is a natural sugar that contains glucose and fructose in equal amounts. We find sucrose in honey and fruits as well as in table sugar. Original corn syrup is just glucose; *high fructose corn syrup* is a sweetener that is made by food processors using regular corn syrup and is approximately one-half glucose and one-half fructose. High fructose corn syrup is very inexpensive to produce and it helps retain moisture in baked products; thus, it is widely used in processed foods.

Honey is a combination of glucose, fructose, and sucrose and is a little sweeter-tasting than table sugar. A relative newcomer to the sweetener market is agave nectar; it is *made* from several types of agave plants grown in Mexico. Agave nectar is not a naturally occurring sugar; the starch from the agave plant is heat-treated to break it into fructose and glucose—you might see "blue agave" nectar in your grocery store. Agave nectar is sweeter than sugar or honey and contains more fructose than glucose.

We could go on and on about the different forms of sugar, but suffice it to say, sugar in and of itself, regardless which of the above forms it comes in, gives us calories in the form of carbohydrates but not much else. Over the past thirty years, as our waistlines have increased, we can definitely point to an increase in added sugars as something that has changed in our diets and the diets of our kids. We are all drinking more sugar-sweetened beverages and fruit juices and eating higher amounts of sugar in processed foods.

Fiber comes from plant foods. There are two types: soluble and insoluble. Soluble fiber is absorbed from our intestine and has been shown to help lower our cholesterol levels; common sources are oats, fruits, and vegetables. Insoluble fiber is not absorbed from our intestine and is very important for keeping our bowels moving—since it is not absorbed, we do not get any calories from it. Common sources of insoluble fiber are the bran in wheat, brown rice, and some of the fiber in fruits and vegetables. Keeping our fiber intake high (both soluble and insoluble) helps us to feel full and is very important when we are trying to decrease calorie intake. We are less apt to have the desire for excess sugar if the sugar we eat comes with fiber (e.g., a piece of fruit instead of a glass of fruit juice).

Eating our complex carbohydrates in the form of whole grains and high fiber, starchy vegetables, and legumes is the healthiest way to get our carbohydrates and the majority of our calories. This also helps prevent some gastrointestinal diseases, such as diverticulosis.

⦿ ⦿ ⦿ ⦿ ⦿ ⦿ ⦿ ⦿ ⦿ ⦿ ⦿ ⦿ ⦿

Fat contains 9 calories per gram (for reference, one teaspoon of *any kind of oil* contains 4.44 gm of fat and 40 calories). Fats come in several varieties—polyunsaturated oils (e.g., corn oil, safflower oil, soy oil, canola oil), all liquid at room temperature and in the refrigerator; monounsaturated oils (olive oil, peanut oil, walnut oil, fish oil), liquid at room temperature but solid in the refrigerator; saturated fat (butter, lard, much of the fat in beef), naturally occurring fats that are solid at room temperature; and trans fats (stick margarines, shortening, the fat often added to commercial baked products and used for commercial fried foods). These trans fats started out unsaturated but had hydrogen added to them to make them more stable and solid at room temperature. Trans fats do not go rancid as fast as polyunsaturated or monounsaturated fats, and they can be heated to higher temperatures without burning (great for deep fat fryers at restaurants, but not good for your arteries!).

Polyunsaturated and many monounsaturated fats are high in essential fatty acids that are required nutrients for us. Both polyunsaturated and monounsaturated fats have been shown to have beneficial effects on our heart health. These fats include canola, corn, safflower, olive, flaxseed, almond, grapeseed, and other oils from vegetables, nuts, seeds, and grains as well as the oil in seafood (salmon, halibut, mackerel, tuna, etc.). Saturated fats and even more so trans fats contribute to high blood cholesterol levels.

Contrary to popular belief, the percentage of fat in our diet has not increased over the past fifty years, but our total fat intake has increased as we increased our total calorie intake. The use of trans fats has increased as we have eaten more processed foods. Current thinking is that we should be eating a moderate amount of healthy fats; limiting saturated fats and avoiding trans fats; and decreasing our sugar and total caloric intake.

●　●　●　●　●　●　●　●　●　●　●　●　●　●　●

Protein contains a little over 4 calories per gram. For reference, meats are very high in protein; one ounce of meat contains approximately 7 grams of protein, which contributes 30 calories; the rest of the calories come from fat, which varies depending on type and cut of meat. In the United States and many Western countries, protein makes up a much bigger proportion of calories than necessary.

Because of relatively high energy needs, typically active children between one and three years of age need only about 5 to 6 percent of their calories from protein—the 23-pound one-year-old needs only 13 grams of protein per day; that is 52 calories from protein out of a total requirement for 840 calories per day. The 31-pound three-year-old needs only 15 grams of protein per day; that is 60 calories from protein out of a total requirement of 1,300 calories per day.

The fast-growing, moderately active, 112-pound, 5-foot 4½-inch fourteen-year-old boy needs about 44 grams of protein, which is only 7 percent of his total energy needs of 2,470 calories per day. Some recent research suggests that very active teenage athletes need about 50 percent more protein than their less active peers, but they also need more calories—if our fourteen-year-old boy was very active (e.g., sports practices for two hours every day plus games once or twice per week), he would need about 61–62 grams of protein per day, and his energy needs would climb to about 3,300 calories per day; protein would make up 7.5 percent of his total energy needs.

My experience is that parents worry far too much about their kids getting enough protein. A typical, moderately active 130-pound adult woman needs about 2,000 calories each day and only 48 grams of protein, which is about 10 percent of her total calorie needs. A typical, moderately active 155-pound adult man needs about 2,500 calories and only 56 grams of protein, which is about 8 percent of total calorie needs. Children and adults typically more than meet their protein needs if they are meeting their calorie needs.

We all need to get our energy from a balance between carbohydrates, protein, and fat. Young children, under two years, need a higher level of fat than older children and adults.

Depending on our cultural heritage, we may eat more of one type of calorie than another; but groups of people who eat high levels of vegetables, legumes, nuts, whole grains, and fish and smaller amounts of meats and dairy products have been shown to have lower rates of obesity, heart disease, and many cancers than those of us living in meat- and cheese-loving cultures. Small amounts of animal foods go a long way toward meeting our needs for iron, zinc, B vitamins, and calcium—we do not need to eat large amounts to be healthy.

Nutrition and Lifestyle References for Families

http://www.eatright.org/public

This is the public page of the American Dietetic Association's website. It is linked to a wide array of information on nutrition for children, including dealing with weight issues. The American Dietetic Association is the credentialing agency for Registered Dietitians throughout the United States and maintains very high standards for the information it produces and references.

http://www.letsmove.gov

First Lady Michelle Obama's website for dealing with the pediatric obesity epidemic gives practical ideas on implementing healthy eating and incorporating physical activity into the lives of our kids.

http://www.brightfuturesforfamilies.org/home.shtml

A website devoted to improving health of children; it includes information on general parenting, family dynamics, kids' health and development, nutrition, physical activity, and much more.

http://www.choosemyplate.gov

A government website that gives detailed information about food and activity needs for individuals of all ages. This also includes interactive tools, which can be used to determine an individual's nutritional needs based on age, weight, height, and gender. The "foodtracker" can be used to enter daily food intake and physical activity and get a calculation of nutrient intake and how it lines up with needs.

http://www.ellynsatter.com

Ellyn Satter has written many very practical books on feeding children and families: *Child of Mine: Feeding with Love and Good Sense* (Bull Publishing Company, 2000); *How to Get Your Kid to Eat ... But Not Too Much* (Bull Publishing

Company, 1987); *Secrets of Feeding a Healthy Family* (Kelcy Press, 1999); and *Your Child's Weight: Helping without Harming, Birth Through Adolescence* (Kelcy Press, 2005). Her website includes a wealth of information on feeding children and dealing with feeding problems (e.g., picky eaters); it also has links to each of her books and her newsletter.

http://www.sleepforkids.org/html/sheet.html

This website gives information on how much sleep our kids need, and practical advice on how to get our kids to sleep.

References

References to books and articles containing the scientific research on which the text is based are listed in the order in which the topic is discussed in each chapter.

Introduction

Ogden J, Clementi C. "The Experience of Being Obese and the Many Consequences of Stigma," *Journal of Obesity* (2010). Online article at http://nebi.nlm.nih.gov/pubmed/20721360.

Hayden MJ, Dixon ME, Dixon JB, Playfair J, O'Brien PE. "Perceived Discrimination and Stigmatisation Against Severely Obese Women: Age and Weight Loss Make a Difference," *Obesity Facts* 3 (Feb. 2010): 7–14.

Farrow CV, Tarrant M. "Weight-based Discrimination, Body Dissatisfaction and Emotional Eating: The Role of Perceived Social Consensus," *Psychology Health* 24 (Nov. 2009): 1021–1034.

Andreyeva TL, Puhl RM, Brownell KD. "Changes in Perceived Weight Discrimination Among Americans, 1995–1996 Through 2004–2006," *Obesity* 16 (May 2008): 1129–1134.

O'Brien KS, Latner JD, Halberstadt J, Hunter JA, Anderson J, Caputi P. "Do Antifat Attitudes Predict Antifat Behaviors?" *Obesity* 16 (Nov. 2008): S87–S92.

Pomeranz JL. "A Historical Analysis of Public Health, the Law, and Stigmatized Social Groups: The Need for Both Obesity and Weight Bias Legislation," *Obesity* 16 (Nov. 2008): S93–S103.

Hearst D. "Can't They Like Me as I Am? Psychological Interventions for Children and Young People with Congenital Visible Disfigurement," *Developmental Neurorehabilitation* 10 (2007): 105–112.

Puhl R, Brownell KD. "Bias, Discrimination, and Obesity," *Obesity Research* 9 (Dec. 2001): 788–805.

Hill AJ, Silver EK. "Fat, Friendless and Unhealthy: 9-Year-Old Children's Perception of Body Shape Stereotypes," *International Journal of Obesity Related Metabolic Disorders* (June 19, 1995): 423–430.

Eliason MJ. "Cleft Lip and Palate: Developmental Effects," *Journal of Pediatric Nursing* 6 (April 1991): 107–113.

Wang Y, Bedoun MA. "The Obesity Epidemic in the United States—Gender, Age, Socioeconomic, Racial/Ethnic, and Geographic Characteristics: A Systematic Review and Meta-Regression Analysis," *Epidemiologic Reviews* 29 (2007): 6 28.

Jacobson MS. "Medical Complications and Comorbidities of Pediatric Obesity," in Sothern MS, Gordon ST, vonAlmen TK, editors. *Handbook of Pediatric Obesity: Clinical Management.* Taylor and Francis Group, 2006. pp. 31–38.

Agras WS, Hammer LD, McNicholas F, Kraemer HC. "Risk Factors for Childhood Overweight: A Prospective Study from Birth to 9.5 years," *Journal of Pediatrics* 145 (July 2004): 20–25.

1 : The "Hows" of Eating

Ollins BY, Belue RZ, Francis LA. "The Beneficial Effect of Family Meals on Obesity Differs by Race, Sex and Household Education: The National Survey of Children's Health, 2003—2004," *Journal of the American Dietetic Association* 110 (Sept. 2010): 1335–1339.

Rovner AJ, Mehta SN, Haynie D, Robinson E, Pound HJ, Butler DA, Laffel LM, Nansel TR. "Perceived Benefits, Barriers and Strategies of Family Meals among Children with Type 1 Diabetes Mellitus and Their Parents: Focus-Group Findings," *Journal of the American Dietetic Association* 110 (Sept. 2010): 1302–1306.

Fulkerson JA, Story M, Neumark-Sztainer D, Rydell S. "Family Meals: Perceptions of Benefits and Challenges among Parents of 8- to 10-Year-Old Children," *Journal of the American Dietetic Association* 108 (April 2008): 706–709.

Wansink B, Van Ittersum K. "Portion Size Me: Downsizing Our Consumption Norms," *Journal of the American Dietetic Association* 107 (July 2007): 1103–1106.

Gable S, Chang Y, Krull JL. "Television Watching and Frequency of Family Meals Are Predictive of Overweight Onset and Persistence in a National Sample of School-Aged Children," *Journal of the American Dietetic Association* 107 (Jan. 2007): 53–61.

Nicklas TA, Morales M, Linares A, Yang SJ, Baranowski T, De Moor C, Berenson G. "Children's Meal Patterns Have Changed over a 21-Year Period: The Bogalusa Heart Study," *Journal of the American Dietetic Association* 104 (May 2004): 753–761.

American Academy of Pediatrics Committee on Nutrition, "Prevention of Pediatric Overweight and Obesity," *Pediatrics* 112 (Aug. 2003): 424–430.

Neumark-Sztainer D, Hannan PJ, Story M, Croll J, Perry C. "Family Meal Patterns: Associations with Sociodemographic Characteristics and Improved Dietary Intake among Adolescents," *Journal of the American Dietetic Association* 103 (March 2003): 317–322.

Nicklas TA, Yang SJ, Baranowski T, Zakeri I, Berenson G. "Eating Patterns and Obesity in Children: The Bogalusa Heart Study," *American Journal of Preventative Medicine* 25 (July 2003): 9–16.

Neumark-Sztainer D, Story M, Perry C, Casey MA. "Factors Influencing Food Choices of Adolescents: Findings from Focus-group Discussions with Adolescents," *Journal of the American Dietetic Association* 99 (Aug. 1999): 929–934, 937.

Satter E. *How to Get Your Kid to Eat . . . But Not Too Much.* Bull Publishing, 1987.

Information on feeding children and dealing with common issues such as "How to Eat." As of November 20, 2010, this information was available online at www.ellynsatter.com.

2: The "Whats" of Eating

Reedy J, Krebs-Smith SM. "Dietary Sources of Energy, Solid Fats and Added Sugars among Children and Adolescents in the United States," *Journal of the American Dietetic Association* 110 (Oct. 2010): 1477–1484.

Kavey R-EW. "How Sweet It Is: Sugar-Sweetened Beverage Consumption, Obesity and Cardiovascular Risk in Childhood," *Journal of the American Dietetic Association* 110 (Oct. 2010): 1456–1460.

Johnson RK, Yon B. "Weighing in on Added Sugars and Health," *Journal of the American Dietetic Association* 110 (Sept. 2010): 1296–1299.

Lustig RH. "Fructose: Metabolic, Hedonic and Societal Parallels with Ethanol," *Journal of the American Dietetic Association* 110 (Sept. 2010): 1307–1321.

Guidelines for healthy eating and nutritional needs, with special pages on children's food and nutrition needs, developed by the U.S. Department of Agriculture. As of May 2011, this information was available online at www .choosemyplate.gov.

Berkey CS, Rockett HRH, Field AE, Gillman MW, Colditz GA. "Sugar-added Beverages and Adolescent Weight Change," *Obesity Research* 12 (2004): 778–788.

Thompson OM, Ballew C, Resnicow K, Must A, Bandini LG, Cyr H, Dietz WH. "Food Purchased Away from Home as a Predictor of Change in BMI Z-Score Among Girls," *International Journal of Obesity Related Metabolic Disorders* 28 (Feb. 2004): 282–289.

James J, Thomas P, Cavan D, Kerr D. "Preventing Childhood Obesity by Reducing Consumption of Carbonated Drinks: Cluster Randomized Controlled Trial," *British Medical Journal* 328 (May 22, 2004): 1237–1242.

American Academy of Pediatrics Committee on Nutrition, "Prevention of Pediatric Overweight and Obesity," *Pediatrics* 112 (Aug. 2003): 424–430.

Ludwig DS, Peterson KE, Gortmaker SL. "Relation between Consumption of Sugar-Sweetened Drinks and Childhood Obesity," *Lancet* 357 (2001): 505–508.

French SA, Story M, Neumark-Sztainer D, Fulkerson JA, Hannan P. "Fast Food Restaurant Use Among Adolescents: Associations with Nutrient Intake, Food Choices and Behavioral and Psychosocial Variables," *International Journal of Obesity* 25 (2001): 1823–1833.

Wardle J, Guthrie C, Sanderson S, Birch L, Plomin R. "Food and Activity Preferences in Children of Lean and Obese Parents," *International Journal of Obesity* 25 (2001): 971–977.

Dennison BA, Rockwell HL, Nichols MJ, Jenkins P. "Children's Growth Parameters Vary by Type of Fruit Juice Consumption," *Journal of the American College of Nutrition* 18 (1999): 346–352.

Ortega RM, Requejo AM, Lopez-Sobaler AM, Quintas ME, Andres P, Redondo MR, Navia B, Lopez-Bonilla MD, Rivas T. "Difference in the Breakfast Habits of Overweight/Obese and Normal Weight School Children," *International Journal for Vitamin and Nutrition Research* 68 (1998): 125–132.

Dennison BA, Rockwell HL, Baker SL. "Excess Fruit Juice Consumption by Preschool-Aged Children Is Associated with Short Stature and Obesity," *Pediatrics* 99 (1997): 15–22.

Summerbell CD, Moody RC, Shanks J, Stock MJ, Geissler C. "Relationship between Feeding Pattern and Body Mass Index in 220 Free-Living People in Four Age Groups," *European Journal of Clinical Nutrition* 50 (1996): 513–519.

3: Kids Are Made to Be Active

Chaput J-P; Klingenberg L, Rosenkilde M, Gilbert J-A, Tremblay A, Sjodin Anders. "Physical Activity Plays an Important Role in Body Weight Regulation," *Journal of Obesity* (2011). Online article ID 360257, doi:10.1155/2011/360257.

Wijga AH, Scholtens S, Bemelmans WJE, Kerkhof M, Koppelman GH, Brunekreef B, Smit HA. "Diet, Screen Time, Physical Activity, and Childhood Overweight in the General Population and in High Risk Subgroups: Prospective Analyses in the PIAMA Birth Cohort," *Journal of Obesity* (2010). Online article ID 423296, available at doi:10.1155/2010/423296.

US Department of Health and Human Services. "Active Children and Adolescents," *Physical Activity Guidelines for Americans*, 2008. ch. 3. Available online as of September 20, 2010, at www.health.gov/paguidelines/guide lines/chapter3.aspx.

Gable S, Chang Y, Krull JL. "Television Watching and Frequency of Family Meals Are Predictive of Overweight Onset and Persistence in a National Sample of School-Aged Children," *Journal of the American Dietetic Association* 107 (Jan. 2007): 53–61.

Council on Sports Medicine and Fitness and Council on School Health. "Active Healthy Living: Prevention of Childhood Obesity through Increased Physical Activity," *Pediatrics* 117 (May 2006): 1834–1842.

Sugimori H, Yoshida K, Izuno T, Miyakawa M, Suka M, Sekine M, Yamagami T, Kagamimori S. "Analysis of Factors That Influence Body Mass Index from Ages 3 to 6 years: A Study Based on the Toyama Cohort Study," *Pediatrics International* 46 (June 2004): 302–310.

American Academy of Pediatrics Committee on Nutrition. "Prevention of Pediatric Overweight and Obesity," *Pediatrics* 112 (Aug. 2003): 424–430.

Berkey CS, Rockett HRH, Gillman MW, Colditz GA. "One-Year Change in Activity and in Inactivity among 10- to 15-Year-Old Boys and Girls: Relationship to Change in Body Mass Index," *Pediatrics* 111 (2003): 836–843.

Bogart N, Steinbeck KS, Baur LA, Brock K, Bermingham MA. "Food, Activity and Family—Environmental vs. Biochemical Predictors of Weight Gain in Children," *European Journal of Clinical Nutrition* 57 (Oct. 2003): 1242–1249.

Francis LA, Lee Y, Birch LL. "Parental Weight Status and Girls' Television Viewing, Snacking and Body Mass Indexes," *Obesity Research* 11 (2003): 143–151.

Storey ML, Forshee RA, Weaver AR, Sansalone WR. "Demographic and Lifestyle Factors Associated with Body Mass Index among Children and Adolescents," *International Journal of Food Science and Nutrition* 54 (2003): 491–503

Janz KF, Levy SM, Burns TL, Torner JC, Willing MC, Warren JJ. "Fatness, Physical Activity and Television Viewing in Children During the Adiposity Rebound Period: The Iowa Bone Development Study," *Preventative Medicine* 35 (2002): 563–71.

Crespo CJ, Smit E, Triano RP, Bartlett SJ, Macera CA, Andersen RD. "Television Watching, Energy Intake and Obesity in US Children," *Archives of Pediatric and Adolescent Medicine* 155 (2001): 360–365.

Dowda M, Ainsworth BE, Addy CL, Saunders R, Riner W. "Environmental Influences, Physical Activity, and Weight Status in 8- to 16-Year-Olds," *Archives of Pediatric and Adolescent Medicine* 155 (2001): 711–717.

Wardle J, Guthrie C, Sanderson S, Birch L, Plomin R. "Food and Activity Preferences in Children of Lean and Obese Parents," *International Journal of Obesity* 25 (2001): 971–977.

Atkin LM, and Davies PS. "Diet Composition and Body Composition in Preschool Children," *American Journal of Clinical Nutrition* 72 (2000): 15–21.

Dietz WH, Gortmaker SL. "Do We Fatten Our Children at the Television Set? Obesity and Television Viewing in Children and Adolescents," *Pediatrics* 75 (1985): 807–812.

4: Teaching Kids About Healthy Eating

Germann JN, Kirchenbaum DS, Rich BH. "Child and Parental Self-Monitoring as Determinants of Success in the Treatment of Morbid Obesity in Low-Income Minority Children," *Journal of Pediatric Psychology* 32 (2007): 111–121.

Dietz WH, Robinson TN. "Overweight Children and Adolescents," *New England Journal of Medicine* 352 (May 19, 2005): 2100–2109.

American Academy of Pediatrics Committee on Nutrition. "Prevention of Pediatric Overweight and Obesity," *Pediatrics* 112 (Aug. 2003): 424–430.

5: Kids' Foods, or Just a Way to Market Junk?

American Academy of Pediatrics Committee on Nutrition, "Prevention of Pediatric Overweight and Obesity," *Pediatrics* 112 (Aug. 2003): 424–430.

Spear BA. "Adolescent Growth and Development," *Journal of the American Dietetic Association* 102 (March 2002): S23–S29.

6: Help for Picky Eaters

Cooke L, Carnell S, Wardle J. "Food Neophobia and Mealtime Food Consumption in 4–5-Year-Old Children," *International Journal of Behavioral Nutrition and Physical Activity* 3 (July 2006): 14–20.

Satter E. *How to Get Your Kid to Eat . . . But Not Too Much.* Bull Publishing, 1987.

7: What Should Parents Be Eating?

Francis LA, Birch LL. "Maternal Weight Status Modulates the Effects of Restriction on Daughters' Eating and Weight," *International Journal of Obesity* 29 (Aug. 2005): 942–949.

Bogart N, Steinbeck KS, Baur LA, Brock K, Bermingham MA. "Food, Activity and Family—Environmental vs. Biochemical Predictors of Weight Gain in Children," *European Journal of Clinical Nutrition* 57 (Oct. 2003): 1242–1249.

Davison KK, Birch LL. "Obesogenic Families: Parents' Physical Activity and Dietary Intake Patterns Predict Girls' Risk of Overweight," *International Journal of Obesity* 26 (2002): 1186–1193.

Davison KK, Birch LL. "Child and Parent Characteristics as Predictors of Change in Girls' Body Mass Index," *International Journal of Obesity Related Metabolic Disorders* 25 (Dec. 2001): 1834–1842.

Davison KK, Birch LL. "Weight Status, Parent Reaction and Self-Concept in Five-Year-Old Girls," *Pediatrics* 107 (2001): 46–53.

Wardle J, Guthrie C, Sanderson S, Birch L, Plomin R. "Food and Activity Preferences in Children of Lean and Obese Parents," *International Journal of Obesity* 25 (2001): 971–977.

Hood MY, Moore LL, Sundarajan-Ramamurti A, Singer M, Cupples LA, Ellison RC. "Parental Eating Attitudes and the Development of Obesity in Children, the Framingham Children's Study," *International Journal of Obesity* 24 (2000): 1319–1325.

Cutting TM, Fisher JO, Grimm-Thomas K, Birch LL. "Like Mother, Like Daughter: Familial Patterns of Overweight Are Mediated by Mothers' Dietary Disinhibition," *American Journal of Clinical Nutrition* 69 (1999): 608–613.

Johnson SL, Birch LL. "Parents' and Children's Adiposity and Eating Style," *Pediatrics* 94 (1994): 653–661.

8: My Child's Weight Is Out of Control—What Should I Do?

Ford AL, Bergh C, Sodersten P, Sabin MA, Hollinghurst S, Hunt LP, Shield JPH. "Treatment of Childhood Obesity by Retraining Eating Behavior: Randomized Controlled Trial," *British Medical Journal* 340 (2010). Online article ID b5388, 2010, available at doi:10.1136/bmj.b5388.

American Dietetic Association. *Healthy Habits for Healthy Kids: A Nutrition and Activity Guide for Parents.* As of September 26, 2010, this information was available online at www.wellpoint.com/healthy_parenting/index.html.

Webber L, Hill C, Cooke L, Carnell S, Wardle J. "Associations between Child Weight and Maternal Feeding Styles Are Mediated by Maternal Perceptions and Concerns," *European Journal of Clinical Nutrition* 64 (March 2010): 259–265.

Barlow SE, Expert Committee. "Expert Committee Recommendations Regarding the Prevention, Assessment and Treatment of Child and

Adolescent Overweight and Obesity: Summary Report," *Pediatrics* 120 (Dec 19, 2007): S164–S192.

Germann JN, Kirschenbaum DS, Rich BH. "Child and Parental Self-Monitoring as Determinants of Success in the Treatment of Morbid Obesity in Low-Income Minority Children," *Journal of Pediatric Psychology* 32 (2007): 111–121.

Wansink B, Van Ittersum, K. "Portion Size Me: Downsizing Our Consumption Norms," *Journal of the American Dietetic Association* 107 (July 2007): 1103–1106.

Golan M. "Parents as Agents of Change in Childhood Obesity—From Research to Practice," *International Journal of Pediatric Obesity* 1 (2006): 66–67.

American Dietetic Association Position Paper. "Position of the American Dietetic Association: Individual-, Family-, School-, and Community-Based Interventions for Pediatric Overweight," *Journal of the American Dietetic Association* 106 (June 2006): 925–945.

Council on Sports Medicine and Fitness and Council on School Health. "Active Healthy Living: Prevention of Childhood Obesity through Increased Physical Activity," *Pediatrics* 117 (May 2006): 1834–1842.

Dietz WH, Robinson TN. "Overweight Children and Adolescents," *New England Journal of Medicine* 352 (May 19, 2005): 2100–2109.

Ebbeling CB, Sinclair KB, Pereirra MA, Garcia-Lago E, Feldman HA, Ludwig DS. "Compensation for Energy Intake from Fast Food Among Overweight and Lean Adolescents," *Journal of the American Medical Association* 291 (June 16, 2004): 2828–2833.

Golan M, Crow S. "Parents are Key Players in the Prevention and Treatment of Weight-related Problems," *Nutrition Reviews* 62 (Jan. 2004): 39–50.

Giammettei J, Blix G, Marshah HH, Wollitzer AO, Tetttitt DJ. "Television Watching and Soft Drink Consumption: Associations with Obesity in 11- to 13-Year-Old School Children," *Archives of Pediatric and Adolescent Medicine* 157 (2003): 882–886.

Boutelle K, Neumark-Sztainer D, Story M, Resnick M. "Weight Control Behaviors Among Obese, Overweight and Non-Overweight Adolescents," *Journal of Pediatric Psychology* 27 (2002): 531–540.

Davison KK, Birch LL. "Processes Linking Weight Status and Self-Concept Among Girls from Ages 5 to 7 years," *Developmental Psychology* 38 (2002): 735–748.

Davison KK, Birch LL. "Weight Status, Parent Reaction and Self-Concept in Five-Year-Old Girls," *Pediatrics* 107 (2001): 46–53.

Lee Y, Mitchell DC, Smiciklas-Wright H, Birch LL. "Diet Quality, Nutrient Intake, Weight Status and Feeding Environments of Girls Meeting or Exceeding Recommendations for Total Dietary Fat of the American Academy of Pediatrics," *Pediatrics* 107 (2001): e95. Available online as of November 20, 2010, at www.pediatrics.org/cgi/content/full/107/6/e95.

Berkey CS, Rockett HRH, Field AE, Gillman MW, Frazier AL, Camargo CA, Colditz GA. "Activity, Dietary Intake and Weight Changes in a Longitudinal Study of Preadolescent and Adolescent Boys and Girls," *Pediatrics* 105 (2000): 1–9.

9: What Does Getting Enough Sleep Have to Do with My Child's Weight?

Darukhanavala A, Pannain S. "Sleep and Obesity in Children and Adolescents," in Bagchi D, editor. *Global Perspectives on Childhood Obesity*. Elsevier, 2011. pp. 167–182.

Bell JF, Zimmerman FJ. "Shortened Nighttime Sleep Duration in Early Life and Subsequent Childhood Obesity," *Archives of Pediatric and Adolescent Medicine* 164 (Sept. 2010): 840–845.

Leproult R, Vancauter E. "Role of Sleep and Sleep Loss in Hormonal Release and Metabolism," *Endocrine Development* 17 (2010): 11–21.

Neighmond P. "Impact of Childhood Obesity Goes Beyond Health," National Public Radio, July 28, 2010. Available online as of September 9, 2010, at www.npr.org.

Liou YM, Liou T-H, Chang L-C. "Obesity Among Adolescents: Sedentary Leisure Time and Sleeping as Determinants," *Journal of Advanced Nursing* 66 (June 2010): 1246–1256.

Lyytikainen P, Lalukka T, Lahelma E, Rahkonen O. "Sleep Problems and Major Weight Gain: A Follow-Up Study," *International Journal of Obesity* (June 8, 2010). Available online at doi:10.1038/ijo.2010.113.

Magee CA, Huang X-F, Iverson DC, Caputi P. "Examining the Pathways Linking Chronic Sleep Restriction to Obesity," *Journal of Obesity* (2010). Online article ID 821710, available at doi:10.1155/2010/821710, 2010.

National Sleep Foundation. "How Much Sleep Do We Really Need?" Available online as of October 11, 2010, at www.sleepfoundation.org/article /how-sleep-works/how-much-sleep-do-we-really-need.

National Sleep Foundation. "Ideas for getting our kids to sleep well, and activities to teach our kids the importance of sleep." Available online as of October 15, 2010, at www.sleepforkids.org.

Patel SR. "Reduced Sleep as an Obesity Risk Factor," *Obesity Reviews* 10 (Nov. 10, 2009): S61–S68.

Patel SR, Hu FB. "Short Sleep Duration and Weight Gain: A Systematic Review," *Obesity* 16 (March 2008): 643–653.

Tikotzky L, De Amrcas G, Har-Toov J, Dollberg S, Bar-Haim Y, Sadeh A. "Sleep and Physical Growth in Infants During the First 6 Months," *Journal of Sleep Research* 29 (March 2010): 103—110.

Shaikh WA, Patel M, Singh SK. "Sleep Deprivation Predisposes Gujarati Indian Adolescents to Obesity," *Indian Journal of Community Medicine* 34 (July 2009): 192–194.

Breus MJ. "Guidelines for Your Child's Bedtime; How to Make It Easier for Your Child (and You!) to Get Sound Sleep," entry on WebMD. Available online at http://children.webmd.com/guide/guidelines-for-your-childs-bedtime.

Sugimori H, Yoshida K, Izuno T, Miyakawa M, Suka M, Sekine M, Yamagami T, Kagamimori S. "Analysis of Factors That Influence Body Mass Index from Ages 3 to 6 years: A Study Based on the Toyama Cohort Study," *Pediatrics International* 46 (June 2004): 302–310.

10: A Word to the Wise About Eating Disorders

Enten RS, Golan M. "Parenting Styles and Eating Disorder Pathology," *Appetite* 52 (2009): 784–787.

Schwimmer JB. "Psychosocial Considerations During Treatment," in Sothern

MS, Gordon ST, vonAlmen TK, editors. *Handbook of Pediatric Obesity: Clinical Management.* Taylor and Francis Group, 2006. pp. 55–65.

Sturdevant MS, Spear BA. "Adolescent Psychosocial Development," *Journal of the American Dietetic Association* 102 (March 2002): S3–S31.

Varner L. *Nutrition Therapy for Patients with Eating Disorders.* Wolf Rinke Associates, Inc., 2003. pp. 117–120.

11: How Environment and Genetics Have Created an Obese Society

Beck M. "Eating to Live or Living to Eat," *Wall Street Journal,* July 13, 2010, pp. D1– D7.

Carnell S, Wardle J. "Appetitive Traits in Children: New Evidence for Associations with Weight and a Common, Obesity-associated Genetic Variant," *Appetite* 53 (2009): 260–263.

Carnell S, Wardle J. "Symposium on 'Behavioral Nutrition and Energy Balance in the Young' Appetitive Traits and Child Obesity: Measurement, Origins and Implications for Intervention," *Proceedings of the Nutrition Society* 67 (2008): 343–355.

Stopeckel LE, Weller RE, Cook EW, Twieg DB, Knowlton RC, Cox JE. "Widespread Reward-System Activation in Obese Women in Response to Pictures of High-Calorie Foods," *NeuroImage* 41 (2008): 636–647.

Rothemund Y, Preuschhof C, Bohner G, Bauknecht H-C, Klingebiel R, Flor H, Klapp B. "Differential Activation of the Dorsal Stiatum by High-Calorie Visual Food Stimuli in Obese Individuals," *NeuroImage* 37 (2007): 410–421.

Wansink B, Van Ittersum K. "Portion Size Me: Downsizing Our Consumption Norms," *Journal of the American Dietetic Association* 107 (July 2007): 1103–1106.

Barlow SE, Expert Committee. "Expert Committee Recommendations Regarding the Prevention, Assessment and Treatment of Child and Adolescent Overweight and Obesity: Summary Report," *Pediatrics* 120 (Dec. 19, 2007): S164–S192.

Council on Sports Medicine and Fitness and Council on School Health. "Active Healthy Living: Prevention of Childhood Obesity through Increased Physical Activity," *Pediatrics* 117 (May 2006): 1834–1842.

Jacobson MS. "Medical Complications and Comorbidities of Pediatric Obesity," in Sothern MS, Gordon ST, vonAlmen TK, editors. *Handbook of Pediatric Obesity: Clinical Management*. Taylor and Francis Group, 2006. pp. 31–38.

Loos RJF, Rankinen T. "Gene-Diet Interactions on Body Weight Changes," *Journal of the American Dietetic Association* 105 (May 2005): S29–S34.

Davison KK, Birch LL. "Child and Parent Characteristics as Predictors of Change in Girls' Body Mass Index," *International Journal of Obesity Related Metabolic Disorders* 25 (Dec. 2001): 1834–1842.

Klesges RC, Klesges LM, Eck LH, Shelton ML. "A Longitudinal Analysis of Accelerated Weight Gain in Preschool Children," *Pediatrics* 95 (1995): 126–130.

National Institute of Diabetes, Digestive and Kidney Diseases, National Institutes of Health. Research on the Pima Indians, published in 2002. Available online as of October 11, 2010, at http://diabetes.niddk.nih.gov /dm/pubs/pima/pathfind/pathfind.htm.

12: What About Calories?

Institute of Medicine of the National Academies. "Energy, Part II" in *Dietary Reference Intakes: The Essential Guide to Nutrient Requirements*. National Academies Press, 2006. pp. 82–93.

Acknowledgments

This book would not have been written without coauthor Sue Schumann Warner. Sue's extensive knowledge of the writing and publishing process, her encouragement as I developed the content, and her excellent writing skills helped to put the book together in a form that will be appealing to parents, grandparents, teachers, youth workers, and all other people who love kids.

Elizabeth Stephen, spiritual director and care ministries coordinator at First Presbyterian Church of Bend, Oregon, inspired me with ways to incorporate spiritual health. Laurie Koski, MSW, clinical social worker in Bend, gave many insights into psychological issues around eating and eating disorders. Peggy Solan, RD, friend and pediatric dietitian at Seattle Children's Hospital went through the book with a fine-tooth comb to evaluate content and flow as well as technical grammar and wording issues. Kristi Nix, MD, pediatrician at Mosaic Medical in Bend, Oregon, and Betsy Perry, elementary school teacher and mom, reviewed the manuscript for overall content, readability, and applicability for parents.

My husband, Bob Brydges, has been my biggest supporter throughout the process of writing this book, and throughout my career as a dietitian. He encourages me and helps keep my life in balance. He has read and reread every section of this book and given his honest opinion about what works, what makes sense, and what doesn't. My children, Suzanne and Michael, have also been great supporters, especially by being great recipe testers. The recipes in this book have been developed over many years, and Suzanne and Michael willingly tested most of them and helped to develop and refine them as well.

I am extremely blessed to have a wonderful network of family, friends, coworkers, as well as clients who have encouraged me and let me know that this is a book that could make a difference in the lives and health of children and their families.

About the Authors

Lori S. Brizee is a registered and licensed clinical dietitian and sought-after speaker with more than twenty-five years of experience. She received her bachelor's degree in dietetics from the University of California at Davis and her master's degree in nutritional sciences at the University of Washington, where she focused on nutrition for children with chronic conditions. For the first twenty-three years of her career, she worked primarily in pediatrics, including twenty years as a clinical nutritionist at Seattle Children's Hospital.

Since 2006 she has had a private nutrition consulting practice in Bend, Oregon, where she sees clients of all ages, with a wide variety of nutritional concerns. She writes about nutrition for newspapers and magazines and is a sought-after speaker on nutritional issues. Her website is www.centraloregonnutrition.com.

Lori is involved in Central Oregon efforts to improve the health and well-being of children: "Kids at Heart," a multidisciplinary effort to reduce childhood obesity, and "Healthy Beginnings," an organization that screens infants and young children for health and development concerns in Central Oregon.

Sue Schumann Warner is an award-winning photojournalist and author who writes on topics ranging from social issues, families, finance, and current events to travel and profiles. She has been published in newspapers and magazines throughout the United States, Europe, and Australia, including the *New York Times*, *Reader's Digest*, *New Man*, *Christian Single*, *Home Life*, and *The War Cry*. She is the coauthor of *Honest, Direct, Respectful . . . Three Simple Words That Will Change Your Life*.

Contact the Author

To schedule a speaking engagement or online nutrition consultation with Lori S. Brizee, go to her website: www.centraloregonnutrition.com.

About Paraclete Press

Who We Are

Paraclete Press is a publisher of books, recordings, and DVDs on Christian spirituality. Our publishing represents a full expression of Christian belief and practice—from Catholic to Evangelical, from Protestant to Orthodox.

We are the publishing arm of the Community of Jesus, an ecumenical monastic community in the Benedictine tradition. As such, we are uniquely positioned in the marketplace without connection to a large corporation and with informal relationships to many branches and denominations of faith.

What We Are Doing

Books   Paraclete publishes books that show the richness and depth of what it means to be Christian. Although Benedictine spirituality is at the heart of all that we do, we publish books that reflect the Christian experience across many cultures, time periods, and houses of worship. We publish books that nourish the vibrant life of the church and its people—books about spiritual practice, formation, history, ideas, and customs.

We have several different series, including the best-selling Paraclete Essentials and Paraclete Giants series of classic texts in contemporary English; A Voice from the Monastery—men and women monastics writing about living a spiritual life today; award-winning literary faith fiction and poetry; and the Active Prayer Series that brings creativity and liveliness to any life of prayer.

Recordings   From Gregorian chant to contemporary American choral works, our music recordings celebrate sacred choral music through the centuries. Paraclete distributes the recordings of the internationally acclaimed choir Gloriæ Dei Cantores, praised for their "rapt and fathomless spiritual intensity" by *American Record Guide*, and the Gloriæ Dei Cantores Schola, which specializes in the study and performance of Gregorian chant. Paraclete is also the exclusive North American distributor of the recordings of the Monastic Choir of St. Peter's Abbey in Solesmes, France, long considered to be a leading authority on Gregorian chant.

DVDs   Our DVDs offer spiritual help, healing, and biblical guidance for life issues: grief and loss, marriage, forgiveness, anger management, facing death, and spiritual formation.

Learn more about us at our website:

www.paracletepress.com, or call us toll-free at 1-800-451-5006.